When
I grow
too old
to
dream

Acknowledgements

The editors wish to acknowledge the encouragement and support of the Board of Management of the Alzheimer Society of Victoria. All royalties from the sale of this book will go to support the work of the Society.

Our thanks to all those who have contributed to this book. We have appreciated the willingness of the contributors to let us and the readers of this book into the deep intimacies of their lives.

To our respective partners our special thanks for their patient endurance during the writing and editing of the book.

This book will add to the rich range of experience on Alzheimer's disease and the other dementias. It is our earnest hope that the book may be of some assistance through the awful journey of Alzheimer's disease.

When I grow too old to dream

Coping with Alzheimer's disease

●●●●●●●●●●●●●●●●●●●●●●●●●

Gerry Naughtin and
Terry Laidler

CollinsDove*Publishers*
A Division of HarperCollins*Publishers*

Published by Collins Dove
A division of HarperCollins*Publishers* (Australia) Pty Ltd
22-24 Joseph Street
North Blackburn 3130

First published 1991
American Edition published 1991
Designed by Noniann Cabouret Lier
Typeset in 11/14 Times by Collins Dove Desktop
Printed in Australia by Griffin Press Pty Ltd

The National Library of Australia
Cataloguing-in-Publication Data:

Naughtin, Gerard.
  When I grow too old to dream.

ISBN 1 86371 075 2.

1. Alzheimer's disease — Patients. 2. Presenile dementia —. 3. Alzheimer's disease —
Patients — Family relationships. 4. Presenile dementia — Patients — Family relationships.
I. Laidler, Terry. II Title.

362.196831

Contents

Acknowledgements   ii

Foreword   vii

PART ONE: BACKGROUND

Introduction   1

The medical background to Alzheimer's
    disease by Professor Colin Masters   9

Stages in the progression of Alzheimer's disease   15

PART TWO: THE STORIES

Margaret: A cup of tea and a chat   17

Anne: Nursing my mom   35

Joan: The key word is care   47

Barbara: Looking for the cues   70

Beth: Alzheimer's—my companion of 20 years   83

Bert: My wife, Joyce   98

Ern: Faith and love   115

Judith: 101 ways to make a bed   125

John and Meg: Twenty beers before dinner   137

Pauline and Cathy: A family under pressure   146

Les and Vera: A lot of tears under the shower   151

Robert: My mom, *Mick*   169

PART THREE: DRAWING THE THREADS TOGETHER

Issues for people facing Alzheimer's disease   190

Where to go for help   226

Susannah: Carer support groups   228

Further reading   239

Foreword

This is a book which explores in an intimate and insightful way two of the major fears of many older and middle-aged people in Western societies — losing one's mind, and being admitted to a nursing home. Loss of memory and eventual admission to residential care are inevitable consequences of developing Alzheimer's disease. As society ages increasing numbers of older people, particularly women, are becoming concerned about how to cope with their own declining physical and mental frailty. Families in their turn are becoming anxious about how they can support and assist their parent, grandparent or uncle or aunt who are growing frail.

This book is timely in that it provides information, support and insight to people who have a dementia or have a loved one with a dementing illness. Because a greater number of people are living beyond seventy and particularly eighty years of age, more people are being affected by the disease and so many more families are feeling its impact. This book shares in a very honest way, the experiences of some people with the disease and some carers, and is full of wise advice which will help those families understand and cope with their situation.

Carers will benefit from learning that their feelings of guilt and powerlessness are not unique. How much better it is when feelings of resentment and the grief for the loss of a loved person can be expressed openly.

The major group affected by this disease is made up of women: more women have the disease and the vast majority of carers both paid and unpaid are female. Indeed the issue of the impact on women's lives and employment opportunities of caring for an ageing parent/relative will be a major social and political issue throughout this decade. We must all recognise that community care places heavy burdens on the few who are carers and public authorities must be willing to provide day-care centres and access to longer periods of respite care to prevent burnout and enable carers to maintain other aspects of their personal and professional lives.

This book helps us recognise the extent of role change involved in caring, over a long period of time, for someone with dementia. It will assist readers in understanding the shock and difficulties that this change of roles involves. The previously powerful and/or respected parent is now in the role of the dependant and this requires adjustment, particularly for the carer. The role change for the person with the dementia is often devastating. The process of change from a determined capable person to one who struggles to remember even names is frustrating for the individual. The spouse must face loneliness and distress when the beloved equal has become an often troublesome dependant.

This book will help the process by which greater information to the public will mean that dementia may be accepted as a disease and feelings of guilt and shame modified and, hopefully, eliminated. These stories show that reluctance to seek help is often a characteristic of carers' behaviour and that they must practise the art of being selfishly unselfish and accept the help which recognises their own needs.

Society must accept that dementia is one of the plagues of the modern age and be willing to cope with it. The growth of the Alzheimer Societies in a very short period has shown the need for this self-help organisation and it has a valuable role in spreading knowledge and advice to those most in need of it.

The book, so clearly based on love and concern and full of sound and practical advice, is all the richer because of its reflection of the human spirit. We can all be grateful to the people who have shared their experiences with us.

Betty Marginson
Deputy Chairperson
Victorian Older Persons Consultative Council
21 August 1990

PART ONE

BACKGROUND

Introduction

This book is about human goodness. It tells the stories of people who have dealt or are dealing with Alzheimer's disease and other forms of progressive dementia. They are diseases which develop subtly, but insidiously, and can affect the individual sufferer for up to fifteen years. They are characterised by a gradual loss of intellectual capacity which slowly strips the person of many life skills and of many key ingredients of their own personality. The person persists, but often as a shell of the one they have been and that others have known. The experience is often shattering for both those with the disease and their primary carers.

Given the rate of ageing of the population and the high impact of the dementias, notably Alzheimer's disease, on those over seventy-five, these diseases are likely to have a profound effect on society, both socially and economically, over the next decade.

The disease involves the gradual dismantling of the physical, social and intellectual capacities of the person affected. The people with dementia are themselves often unable to understand the changes in their personality and their own diminishing functions. Such changes are often put down to change of life or late-life menopause for women. For the person with the disease, there is a real struggle to maintain control of their world, to keep a hold on realities they have been able to deal with, automatically, for many years.

Carers have to adjust to living with a very different person from the one with whom they have shared a strong bond. While the physical body of the person is often in fine form, the actual personality and the intellect start to diminish.

Gradually carers see themselves losing a life companion, perhaps the very one they would normally have relied on to get through times as tough as those they see ahead. The person with dementia begins to become physically and emotionally dependent upon the carer.

Because of this dependency, the progress of this disease often raises life-long relationship issues. Behavioural traits of childhood can emerge as the person is seen to revert to uninhibited habits of behaviour learned long ago. Much of social conditioning, and conscience, is lost and the person relies increasingly on more primary responses. Awareness of social sanctions is reduced. Personality and marital or family tensions frequently become exacerbated.

There is often enormous anger and frustration either at a shared lifetime curtailed, or lack of financial opportunity and the frustration of a dependent relationship just at a time when the carer was hoping for a more secure and independent life-style.

The carer must deal with the slow death of the person they have known. Much of the tension and trauma associated with the care of people with dementia relates to changing roles.

Adult children must often take on the parent role with their own parent.

For a couple who have shared a relationship where the male has played a dominant role, the shift when the wife has to take control role in the household, to run the family finances, to make key financial, legal and life choices, often requires significant change at an age when change is most difficult.

For children, decisions such as stopping a parent from driving the car or taking control of the family's finances involves a significant shift in role.

These role changes, combined with poor understanding of the disease and its management, often make care and management a difficult and complex function.

The complexities of dealing with a chronic illness are not unique to Alzhemier's disease and the progressive dementias. However, the subtlety of their development, the complexity of the emotional shifts and role changes for both the person affected and their carers is unique. In addition, there is still a degree of stigma associated with the notion of mental disease. This, in part, relates to ignorance and fear of the disease.

Nonetheless, the support, care and management of people with dementia can challenge, threaten and bring out the very best and worst in carers.

The people who have contributed to the book come from diverse backgrounds. Most of the stories in it are the stories of carers; a couple of the contributors themselves suffer from memory loss and dementia. Most of the carers are family members; professional carers reflect on their experience as well. Most care for people with dementia caused by Alzheimer's disease, but there are also stories about people with Korsakoff's psychosis and multiple infarct dementia. We hope that the diversity of contributors will serve to give breadth to the understanding of what it is like to care for a person with dementia.

The Editors

Both the editors have had direct experience of the disease. Gerry's father developed Alzheimer's disease some ten years ago. For the first few years, there were only small changes: forgetfulness about the date or about events, the need for reminders about certain domestic tasks. His forgetfulness was put down to adjustments to retirement or part of the ageing process. However, it developed and was noticed by his wife because of their shared day-to-day life. Having worked in the field of care for the aged for some time and recognising the symptoms, Gerry thought it would be relatively straightforward to raise the matter with his mother. She, in her turn felt the need to protect, to look after her partner of a life time, not to show the kids (all of whom were mature adults with professional backgrounds). The maintenance of the father's selfesteem and public dignity was seen to be of paramount importance.

Gerry's father died with bowel cancer two years ago. While, professionally, as a social worker, Gerry had a good background knowledge of dementia, the actual experience of supporting his mother and caring for his father is, by his account, the most emotionally devastating experience of his life to date.

Gerry now works with the Alzheimer Society of Victoria as its Executive Director. He oversees part of the support network often referred to by contributors to the book.

Terry worked for many years as a Catholic priest. Many of the older people who were part of his communion round, and those who cared for them, were dealing with dementia day by day. As a trained psychologist, he has counselled carers whose guilt, anxiety and depression added burdens to the practical loads they had taken on. A stint in that part of the Health Department which dealt with Nursing Homes, hostels and older people's services, where he worked with Gerry, has given him some appreciation of the breadth of human endeavour that goes into the care of people suffering from dementia.

More recently, Terry has also had to cope with the impact of Alzheimer's disease close to home. His partner's mother is suffering from dementia. He has experienced the powerlessness of wanting to help, but never quite knowing how best to support. He has been frustrated by the inadequacy of the formal support networks that he thought he knew so well. He knows the strains placed on his partner by the changing relationship at home, and the way that displaced frustration has in turn strained their relationship.

Both of us were touched and moved by the stories that are the substance of this book because we had laughed and cried at many situations similar to those described.

The concept behind the book

There are many text and reference books available about Alzheimer's and related diseases. However, there is little material that presents the experience through the eyes of affected persons and their carers. Similarly, much has been written about coping with death and grieving and much has been developed in the provision of more humane approaches to dying through palliative care programs. However, little of this is relevant to the experience of the person with the disease or the reaction of the family.

Often, reference materials take the form of the professional telling carers what to do, and how to do it.

This book takes a different tack. It is written to lay out both the experience of the disease by the person affected as well as the experience of the person primarily responsible for his or her care.

It begins with some basic factual information about Alzheimer's disease and some tables which help one to understand its progress. These are provided for context.

The body of the book has been developed around a biographical theme using people's own stories to try and illustrate the distinctive and often devastating nature of this disease. The stories illustrate the diverse ways in which people cope with the disease.

It presents their lives and their reactions to the disease in their own terms. It offers readers the opportunity to understand the disease through their lives, through their hopes and through their frustrations.

Its conceptual or theoretical framework is simple. It is borrowed, in part, from a structure used by Susan Kelly and Prasuna Reddy in their book about coping with life crises, *Outrageous Fortune* (Allen & Unwin/Haley, Sydney, 1989).

Contributors were asked to describe in their own words their experience in dealing with Alzheimer's disease and other progressive dementias using a set of twelve questions as a guide. They were also invited to consider issues and questions which are not raised in the set of questions provided, but which had been particularly relevant to them in coping with Alzheimer's disease.

The set of questions is shown below:

THE BEGINNINGS:

1 How and when did you first start to be aware that there was a problem? What did you think the problem was? What events did you see in a new light?

2 Describe how the disease progressed. What changes did you experience in yourself (e.g. health, self-esteem) at that time?

3 What changes did you experience in your relationships with others?

ACTUALLY COPING:

4 What did you find particularly hard to cope with (e.g. physical symptoms in yourself such as insomnia, stomach upset, headaches; disturbing thoughts; managing your feelings; uncertainty about the future; making sense of what was happening; etc.)?

5 What emotions do you most recall experiencing at different stages (e.g. fear, anger, guilt, sadness, loneliness, confusion, rejection, etc.)?

6 What did you do at different stages to cope with the difficulties or other stresses you were experiencing? Coping can include a wide array of strategies which can occur separately or together. For example, one can:

   • try to understand the situation in terms of past experiences

- try to find a general purpose or pattern of meaning in the course of events
- focus on something good that might come out of the difficulties one is experiencing
- deny or minimise the seriousness of what is occurring
- seek information from books, friends, counsellors, about the disease and ways of handling it
- seek support from friends, family or others who may or may not have had to cope with Alzheimer's disease themselves
- change something about oneself or the situation in which one finds oneself to meet certain demands (e.g. getting more sleep, taking tranquillisers, taking up heavy drinking or smoking, taking up rigorous exercise, going to self-development sessions, setting a new timetable, etc.)
- make efforts to maintain hope, and control one's emotions
- openly vent one's feelings
- give up and accept one's fate
- withdraw into oneself, avoid family and friends
- throw oneself into other areas of activity.

LONG TERM CHANGES:

7 Describe how your patterns of coping changed over time (e.g. from when you first confronted the disease, to when you became aware of its implications, from when changes in behaviour were minimal to when they became marked, right up to the present).

8 How effectively would you say you have coped? Do you think you have managed as well as you might have? What have you learned from your experience to date that might help you in other ways?

9 How has dealing with Alzheimer's disease changed you? How has it changed your relationships with others? Has it been a major turning point for you? Or was it just one of the many difficulties you have had to manage throughout your lifetime?

10 Has coping with Alzheimer's disease changed your values, your philosophy of life, your view of people? (e.g. Are you more or less trusting now? Do you live more for the present? Are you a better planner? Do you put your time into different pursuits or different relationships now than before you had to deal with Alzheimer's disease? Have you become more religious or more spiritually oriented?)

11 If you had to choose one thing, person, insight or strategy that helped you confront Alzheimer's disease, what would that be? Please say why.

12 Finally, if you had your time again, what would you do differently if you had to meet exactly the same situation? Why?

The editors have tried in the final chapter to draw common threads from the stories of contributors. In some ways, this is less important and less telling than the stories themselves. However, it is offered in the hope that it will help to reinforce and pull together major insights of the people who have been courageous enough to tell their stories for others' gain.

The editors also hope that contributors themselves have gained from writing. It seems they may have. Many commented, both in their articles, and privately to the editors, that the experience of putting pen to paper had been extremely beneficial to them, that it had helped in their coping by giving them the chance to pull their thoughts together. Some even suggested that it could be a worthwhile thing for others to do.

The book concludes with some practical reference material, both for sources of information and of practical support.

It is our hope that the enterprise will ease the load of those whose genuine goodness often goes unsung, and whose need for assurance that they are not alone is often of major significance as they manage incredibly well against great odds.

The medical background to Alzheimer's disease

By Colin Masters

Chairman of the Department of Pathology, University of Melbourne, and a leading international researcher into the cause of Alzheimer's disease.

Symptoms and signs

The word, dementia, covers many aspects of disturbed intellect, but it is helpful to convey the idea that in Alzheimer's disease, many varied disturbances of brain function can occur. Usually, the onset of dementia in Alzheimer's disease is insidious and occurs over many months. Most often, the affected person is unaware of any failings, and it is the carer who first notices those lapses in memory or disturbances in behaviour which are out-of-keeping with the usual temperament of the patient. There comes a point where memory loss for recent events begins to interfere with normal daily activities.

Similarly, the gradual loss of intellect (ability to calculate, to manage the household finances, to recognise and remember new and familiar faces) and progressive disorientation in time and space (inability to keep appointments, loss of knowledge of the day of the week, getting lost driving a car or when returning by foot from a shopping trip) are early features of Alzheimer's disease.

Altered behaviour patterns also figure prominently, but these are difficult to categorise in the early stages and often result from a mixed deficit in many areas of intellectual function.

By the time medical attention is sought, it is usually fairly obvious that a serious problem exists, one which the patient is beginning to recognise, and by which depressive symptoms may be generated. The doctor, who may be a general practitioner or specialist (geriatrician, neurologist, psychiatrist) will take a detailed history and examination looking for the causes of dementia that may be treatable. At this time, there is no specific test for Alzheimer's disease — that is, there is no blood test or a biochemical test on cerebrospinal fluid which will identify an Alzheimer's disease sufferer.

In most instances, it is the passage of time which will disclose the real nature of the underlying illness. The doctors in charge of the patient will need to re-assess the evolution of the symptoms and signs at approximately six-month intervals. If there is evidence of a steady decline, this will be an important factor in diagnosis.

Some specialists may order radiological or other tests to help them exclude some treatable causes of dementia. A computerised tomographic (CT) scan may help diagnose blood vessel disease in some cases. In others, a blood test may confirm the presence of a low thyroid gland function.

As the disease progresses, usually over a period of several years, the signs and symptoms become progressively worse. Most areas of brain function can be involved in this process, but the changes most noted are to do with the ability of the patient to communicate and to take care of their personal needs (feeding, toiletry, etc.). While the patient is still able to walk (ambulatory stage of Alzheimer's disease), then disorientation and memory loss combine to cause difficulties with wandering behaviour. Often, ambulant patients need to be restrained within a secure environment. Inevitably, the disease progresses to a point where the patient is bed-fast and requires continual nursing care. Throughout the ambulatory and bed-fast stages, major problems arise with urinary and faecal incontinence — subjects which are dealt with elsewhere in this book.

The Cause of Alzheimer's Disease

If we knew the cause of Alzheimer's disease, we could start to treat the disease specifically, and eventually find a way of preventing it. Unfortunately, no-one knows what causes Alzheimer's disease. This is why we spend all our time and effort in trying to unravel the clues that exist so far.

The major change that we see in the brain of a person who dies from Alzheimer's disease is the accumulation of an abnormal protein (called amyloid) in spaces between cells (plaques) and within cells (neurofibrillary tangles). It appears that this amyloid is damaging the nerve cells, which gradually shrink in size and disappear. Most recent work in this field is directed at finding out how this amyloid protein accumulates in the Alzheimer's diseased brain.

The photomicrograph shows many plaques in the brain tissue of a person with Alzheimer's disease. The biochemical nature of these plaques is central to our understanding of the cause of Alzheimer's disease.

Figure 1 This is a photomicrograph of brain tissue affected with Alzheimer's disease. The larger black spheres are the amyloid plaques which accumulate during the disease process. Between the plaques, the faint outlines of the nerve cells are seen.

The diagram shows schematically the different cells which are associated with the deposition of amyloid protein in the centre of the plaque. These cells (astrocytes and microglia) are reacting to the injury caused by the amyloid protein.

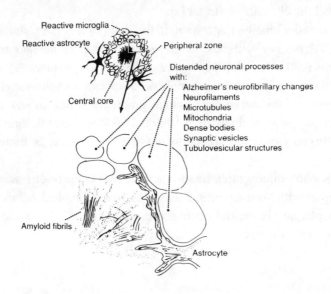

Reactive microglia
Reactive astrocyte
Peripheral zone
Distended neuronal processes with:
Alzheimer's neurofibrillary changes
Neurofilaments
Central core
Microtubules
Mitochondria
Dense bodies
Synaptic vesicles
Tubulovesicular structures
Amyloid fibrils
Astrocyte

Figure 2 This is a diagrammatic sketch of the changes in the amyloid plaque. In the upper part of the figure, reactive cells (microglia and astrocytes) are seen around the periphery of the central core of the amyloid plaque. In the lower figure, some of the changes which occur in the normal surrounding tissue are listed. It is the distension of these neuronal processes which seems to correlate with the disturbances of nerve cell function (dementia) in Alzheimer's disease.

Many studies have taken place in the last thirty years looking for risk factors which might predispose an individual to getting Alzheimer's disease. So far, only three have been identified:
· increasing age;
· family history of disease (genetics);
· Down's Syndrome.
· Let us have a look at these in more detail.
Increasing age as a risk factor This seems to be a constant factor all around the world: the incidence of Alzheimer's disease in-

creases dramatically (exponentially) with increasing age after fifty years. It is true that some Alzheimer's disease cases occur in the fifties and sixties, but most occur after seventy years. There is evidence that the changes in the brain take about thirty years to develop to the point where the patient experiences difficulty. We do not understand the factors that control this age-related phenomenon.

Family history and genetics At least ten per cent of Alzheimer's disease cases occur in families where there is a strong history of other members being affected. Since Alzheimer's disease affects both males and females, and occurs at a rate of about fifty per cent in each generation of these families, we call this an autosomal dominant form of Familial Alzheimer's disease. We now recognise that the Familial Alzheimer's disease gene is an important factor in determining the onset of disease, and efforts are now being made in many research laboratories to identify this gene. We might eventually be able to control this gene's function. Once the gene is identified, we will also be able to perform genetic counselling and pre-natal diagnosis.

Down's Syndrome and Alzheimer's disease In Down's Syndrome, the changes of Alzheimer's disease occur in every person by the age of thirty years. We now know that the amyloid protein is coded for by a gene on chromosome 21, which is at fault in Down's Syndrome. This provides us with an important clue as to what may be amiss in Alzheimer's disease, but as yet this has not been fully elucidated.

These three risk factors are the sum total of all the applied research to date. Clearly, we have a long way to go. There are many hypotheses and suggestions on what could be in the environment and causing Alzheimer's disease. Some of these (such as aluminium poisoning nor a slow virus infection) are based on evidence derived from experimental models. Other theories have been put forward with very little to back them up. At present, we can only state that neither aluminium or slow virus has been definitely shown to cause Alzheimer's disease. Much more work on these subjects is required.

A Treatment For Alzheimer's Disease

With the heightened awareness regarding Alzheimer's disease, there is much more research being carried out throughout the world. It will be many years before any of this research can be translated into an effective therapy.

While this research is being undertaken, there will be increasing publicity given to proposed new methods of treatment. Each new proposal brings with it a measure of hope that at least a cure for Alzheimer's disease is close at hand. The problem, of course, is that each proposed method of treatment will have to undergo rigorous assessment to see if it really works. Failure to do this means that we run the risk of causing harm to patients with Alzheimer's disease, and creating false hopes in those who care for the Alzheimer's disease victim.

At this time, there is no specific treatment for Alzheimer's disease. The prospect for such a treatment lies firmly with new discoveries made through basic research into the nature and cause of Alzheimer's disease. This is the method that has worked in the past, in treating infectious diseases such as polio and tuberculosis, in reducing the complications of high blood pressure, and in the case of many other life-threatening diseases. It is certainly the method that we are following in our laboratories, and by which we share in the knowledge which is generated world-wide.

There have been some spectacular advances in our understanding of Alzheimer's disease in the last ten years, and to some of these we are pleased to have contributed. But all the signs are that it will be a long hard road before the specific therapy for Alzheimer's disease appears.

In the meantime, we and others are driven forward by the certainty that Alzheimer's disease can be fully understood at a very basic level, and through this understanding a specific therapy will emerge.

Stages in the progression of Alzheimer's disease

To help understand the stories in this book, the tables provided map out a general pattern common to the progressive dementias. They are not meant to describe each individual case in detail, but to give an overview of a general tendency in the way the disease develops.

Behaviours and symptoms at the different stages

STAGE 1: FORGETFULNESS (MILD)

- Increasing forgetfulness identified as a problem
- Changes in personality
- Some disorientation of time, place, speech
- Difficulties with complex problems, planning and decision making
- Some insight into condition:
  anxiety
  denial
  anger
- Difficuties in coping with social situations
- Difficulties for sufferer, carer or family in accepting the disease

STAGE 2: CONFUSION (MODERATE)

- Deterioration in skills of daily living:
  dressing and cooking
  personal hygiene
  financial management

- Personality changes:
  fastidiousness
  jealousy
  aggression
- Deterioration in memory and concentration
- Losing things, wandering
- Disturbed sleep
- Disorientation of time and place
- Strong reliance on primary carer—*clinging behaviour*
- Loss of social limits
- Beginings of incontinence, loss of trust, fear of being afraid
- *Home* a feeling rather than a place

STAGE 3: DEMENTIA (SEVERE)

- Increasing confusion and disorientation
- High levels of agitation and sometimes aggression
- Continual wandering
- Incontinence of urine and/or faeces
- Abnormal body movements
- Finally become immobile, unable to feed oneself; weight loss
- Delusions and hallucinations
- Need to be able to move about and consequent need for security and sometimes restraint

PART TWO

THE STORIES

Margaret: A cup of tea and a chat

My story is written from the perspective of a professional who has worked for many years both in home care services, and in residential care, with people who had dementia and their carers. Looking back over the years, I realise I learned a great deal about the tenacity of carers and the way in which people cope in the most difficult circumstances.

I encountered a person with dementia very early in my career, and learned to my dismay that many of the things I had read in text books, and had been taught in my professional training, did not necessarily apply when I was confronted with how to offer a person with dementia a service they did not ask for, or indeed believe they needed. This was particularly difficult when the person lived alone, and did not have a family member to act on their behalf. I also had difficulty coming to terms with the family member or friend who had requested that I make a home visit to do an assessment, and would then ask me not to tell the person who I was or why I was there.

As a general rule, I was asked to intervene too late, when the situation was at crisis point and the carer or neighbours were at their wits' end. My training had taught me always to offer people choices, to let them decide, and above all never to foster dependence. I soon discovered that these theories did not work so smoothly with people who had dementia.

If I could give some examples from my community care days: the first person I helped place in a special accommodation house walked out the door half an hour after I left her there. When I offered choices to people with dementia, they became even more confused and anxious. Trying to reason with them did not work: they thought I was the one who was being unreasonable.

The cup of tea

The word, assessment, took on a different meaning for me when I was confronted with how to get into the house, particularly if the person lived alone. It was not unusual for me to arrive at a house to find the person either not there or locked inside or outside the house. On the other hand, on some occasions it was too easy to get in when it was quite obvious that the person would have allowed anyone into the house, placing them in danger of being attacked, robbed or exploited. I found that going to the door looking official did not work. I would simply say that so-and-so had sent me, either the doctor or a friend or relative. Unless the person was severely affected by dementia, it was unusual not to be offered a cup of tea.

However, the very fact that I was prepared to have a cup of tea put me in a different category. If the person had a carer who did not want me to tell the person who I was or why I was there, I would ask them to organise a cup of tea as if I were a visitor. I would also ask the carer not to answer the questions for the person. Some carers found this difficult as they were so used to filling in the gaps in the person's memory in order to protect them from the outside world. Before my visit I would also explain to carers that they were not to worry if the person got angry or aggressive with me, as I was after all a visitor to their home who was, as far as the person with dementia was concerned, uninvited. Although the carer had asked me not to say who I was, I would tell the person the truth when they asked. As I was aware of the fact that the person related very much at a feeling level, it put everyone at ease and allowed the assessment to be carried out.

The cup-of-tea situation does several things: it makes the visit more normal; it gives the carer something to do, particularly if they are very anxious; if the person with dementia makes the tea (or tries to), it provides a very quick assessment of their cognitive functioning and co-ordination, vision etc.; over a cup of tea, the person with dementia would produce all sorts of information. (The only problem with this style of assessment is that the assessor puts on weight!)

I was always acutely aware of the high levels of stress experienced by carers in trying to come to terms with the disease, and as the result of their caring role. Their feelings of powerlessness were also evident as they struggled with their loss and lack of control over the way in which the disease was robbing them of the person they knew and loved. In my experience, families suffered the most painful emotions when they had to make a decision about whether or not to relinquish their loved one to long-term care. Faced with this decision, carers across the board experienced the same self-doubts: Were they making the correct decision? Was it the right time to allow the person with dementia to go into care? Had they really done all they could?

In many instances, this decision had been taken out of their hands, either because their own health had broken down or a professional worker made the decision for them.

The professional/compassionate conflict

As a professional worker one of the main struggles for me in working with people with dementia was the one between being professional and being compassionate towards another human being whose future depended on the way in which you perceived them and the way they really were. I will illustrate this with a story of my involvement with an elderly woman.

I met her for the first time in a locked ward of a psychiatric hospital. She had been admitted there because she had been hitch-hiking all around the state trying to get home. She was sitting straight-backed and holding the newspaper as if she were really reading it while people all around her were pacing up and down or calling out. My initial impression was of a sad, aloof woman. However, I travelled with this woman through her journey from leaving the psychiatric hospital until she was finally admitted to a nursing home to end her days. I found it impossible not to get attached to her as I watched her struggle to make sense of a new environment. I was responsible for moving her from the psychiatric hospital to a different type of accommodation. My colleague and I travelled with her back to the old home and were confronted with all of the evidence of what this woman had been.

She had been an exquisite dressmaker. Remnants of the silk she had used over the years were neatly folded away in bags. There was also evidence of the yards and yards of material she had bought while she was in the early stages of her dementia and believed she was still dressmaking. I watched grief overcome this woman when we walked in the garden where her only son had dropped dead while they were both gardening only a few months before. He had been her carer. She was not able to articulate why she was feeling sad but she knew it was associated with the garden.

I observed this woman change from a frightened, sad woman to one who believed she was one of the workers in the residential care facility where she lived. I watched her relinquish her handbag with confidence to her bedroom where she felt it was safe. I was delighted when she and a relative re-established a relationship which had been damaged as the result of her behaviour in the early stages of her dementia. I celebrated Christmas with her. How could I not become attached to her?

I think the main thing I learned as a professional working with people with dementia was that all my text book learning provided me with was a paradigm for things I already knew intuitively. You treat a person with dementia the way you would treat anyone else, as another human being, albeit one who has lost their memory.

Double loss

Carers on the other hand are experiencing two losses, the loss of the person and the loss of their role in connection to that person.

In the intervening thirteen years, I have worked with large numbers of people with dementia and have been involved with carers from all walks of life. I have always been amazed at how different they are in their ability to cope. Some families are able to manage with the most incredible demands placed on them, while others are rendered almost incapable of dealing with the situation as soon as the person exhibits the slightest change in their personality, or behaves in a way that is socially unacceptable to the family.

Some issues which emerged consistently over the years affected the people with dementia at many levels and, subsequently, contributed to whether the carer coped or otherwise with their caring role.

The quality of the relationship between the carer and the person with the dementia prior to the onset of the disease played an important part in the way carers responded to their role. The same applied to the type and degree of assistance carers received from other family members.

How carers were treated by professionals and other workers with whom they came into contact often had a major long-term effect. The way in which both carers and the people with dementia were treated by service providers also played a major part in whether or not the carer was able to cope. The latter depended a great deal on the level of skill and knowledge of dementia of professionals and other workers, and what type of services they had to offer.

The attitudes of neighbours and the amount of support people with dementia living alone received from them and other members of the community were contributing factors with regard to when people with dementia were deemed by their carers to be unsuitable to live alone.

Added to this, my experience has been that it is the exception rather than the rule for families to seek help when the person with dementia is in the early stages of the disease. More often than not, they wait until they can no longer cope before they ask for assistance. In many cases, they see it as an admission of failure to ask for help. In other cases, carers have sought out assistance only to be told that nothing can be done, or to go home and not worry about it.

Another common dilemma for carers is when the person with dementia is so adept at hiding their condition that other family members and even professionals find it hard to believe that there is anything wrong with the person, and wonder why the carer is making such a fuss about the person's behaviour.

In the early stages, the changes are very subtle. Therefore, it is not difficult for people who do not have daily contact with the person with dementia to be fooled. Even during these early stages carers can be feeling their loss acutely: the loss of their own role as spouse, child, friend, and the gradual loss of the competence and personality of the person with dementia. Dealing with the complexity of these issues requires energy that the carer may or may not have. Because of this, workers do need to take a slightly different approach.

After diagnosis

Immediately following diagnosis, carers can and do suffer from shock. Even when they suspect that something is wrong, it is a different matter when they are actually told that the diagnosis is dementia and that nothing can be done. If the diagnosis has been made when the person with dementia is in the early stages of the disease, they can be confused and disoriented one day and rational the next. This is a very unsettling time for carers who often believe during these good days that the person is getting better. It is also an extremely painful time when they see the person slipping away from them while they stand by, powerless to do anything about it. I believe that it is this feeling of powerlessness which has such a profound effect on carers and starts them on the grieving process. This grieving has been called 'the funeral that never ends'. However, I believe it is because, as a society, we do not have a ritual which acknowledges that we can lose a person although they have not died. As a society, we know how to treat physical pain and death. We have difficulty dealing with emotional pain that is not seen to be the result of something tangible, as in this case, with the loss of the person with dementia before they have actually died.

Therefore, carers must be supported and encouraged to discuss this loss and have it affirmed. They must also be helped to understand that what they are feeling is a normal part of grieving. Education about the disease and what the carer might expect in the short term are crucial pieces of information at this stage. I have found that it is also important to discuss fears which carers may have about the hereditary aspects of the disease.

It is important not to saturate the carer with information at this time, as it is a time of very high stress. If the person with dementia is still in the early stages of the disease, they may well be aware of the fact that something is happening to their memory.

It was during this time that I found carers did not want me to tell the people with dementia why I had come to visit them. What I did in these cases was actually tell the person who I was when they asked and say that someone they knew had asked me to visit them.

In the early stages, I think carers also need to consider the legal issues of the situation, particularly with regard to enduring power of attorney, as it may be the last opportunity for the people with dementia to understand what they are signing. It is also useful at this time to explain the reason for some of the behaviours which carers are having difficulty understanding, for example, the repetitive questioning that is part of the short term memory loss. It can be reassuring for carers to be told that the person with dementia is not being difficult, but that the strange behaviour is the result of damage to the person's brain, and that they have a physical condition which is causing the problem. It is often a relief for carers to know that they do not need to be ashamed of the person's condition and that thousands of people in the country are dealing with similar problems.

However, they do need to be assured even if they believe that other people are worse off than they are that they are still entitled to seek help. I encourage them to make plans for a regular break away from their caring role. This can be a big decision, as often in the initial stages the people with dementia may refuse to go to day care or spend some time with another family member because they do not believe that they need someone to supervise them.

Irrespective of how old the person is, they will believe in many cases that they are much younger than they are and refuse to stay at the day care center or some other place 'with these old people'. Their perception of the situation is clouded as the result of the damage to their brain.

It is important that carers and the people with dementia be given time to adjust to their new life situation. Carers may feel guilty about leaving the person, especially if they are refusing to stay.

It is important to explain to the carer that people with dementia may refuse to do a particular thing one week and then be quite happy to consent to do the very same thing the next week. In other words, the refusal to take part in a particular activity is not based on a rational decision. Once the person with dementia feels OK about the place and the people they will most likely settle.

An additional reason why carers should be encouraged to seek help in the early stages is that the caring process may go on for many years. They need help to convince themselves that it is all right to have some time to themselves, that, in the long run, this will make them a better carer and help eliminate some of the stress which is a consequence of caring for people with dementia.

Practical advice

Carers also need to be given practical advice regarding the aids and appliances which are available to assist them in managing some of the behaviours which people with dementia exhibit, and which are regarded as a problem. Carers are all very different and what is considered a problem for one may not worry another.

Some of the more common ones I have encountered are night-time restlessness, incontinence, going out of the house and getting lost, refusing to shower or change their clothes, and not eating. If the person with dementia lives apart from the carer, advice is needed about issues of safety and security, nutrition and the administering of medication. Carers should be given an explanation about the fact that people with dementia have short concentration spans and are easily distracted .

An explanation of some of the basic facts about how the person's brain is affected as the result of the dementia can assist carers to be more understanding and patient, as they realise that the person is not just being difficult. I often needed to explain to a carer that it was a waste of their time and energy to argue with the person with dementia, as they are not able to sustain an argument or to be rational. I find this can benefit both the carer and the person with dementia.

I think it also useful to explain to carers that the person with dementia is not able to alter their behaviour to suit the environment, but that there are many practical things a carer can do to help reduce some of the stress.

Dealing with difficult behaviours

Carers have a variety of levels of coping and some manage very difficult behaviours in ingenious and creative ways. There are however some behaviours that even the most stoical of carers have difficulty with. Some of these include dressing and undressing all day, urinating in unusual places, finger-painting with or wrapping up little parcels of faeces and presenting them to all and sundry at the most inappropriate times.

Accusing the carer of stealing things and telling stories which are not true, especially to other family members and neighbours, are other behaviours which carers find difficult. The latter behaviour can cause family divisions which are very difficult to mend, particularly if one of the other family members is not coping emotionally with the fact that the person has the disease.

Dressing and undressing all day long appears to be a behaviour which is common among women who have dementia. It can be avoided to a certain extent. Locking the cupboard may stop it, but it can also make the person very angry when they find their possessions locked up. A simpler solution I have seen a lot of people adopt is to take most of the clothing out of the wardrobe and leave only a few items for the person to choose from. This should be done when the person is not there. Care should be taken to make sure that old pieces of clothing are left that the person with dementia recognises, even some which are very shabby and need replacing. Although the clothing may appear to us old and not fit to wear, it can be a source of comfort to people with dementia.

Another behaviour which I have noticed carers find hard to deal with is when the person with dementia confabulates, or makes up stories. I believe the TV, which is often used as an activity, actually contributes to this. People with dementia do confuse what is going on in the television with real life. I am not suggesting that carers do not allow the person to watch television if that provides them with a break. I merely want to point out that it can contribute to their telling stories which are not based on reality.

In this range of behaviours, carers may also have to manage catastrophic reactions said to be caused by over-stimulation which places excessive stress on the people with dementia. They have also been attributed to reliving old memories which upset or frightened the person.

Walking with intent, or wandering as it is usually referred to, is another behaviour which causes much fear and distress for carers. Some, but not all, people with dementia have a propensity to go walking late in the afternoon. They are usually going home, home often being a place from the past which may no longer exist. I believe this going home to be a feeling for security and safety at the end of the day.

Therefore, the solution is to respond to the person's need for security and comfort. Many people do this simply with words, reassuring them that they are safe and will be taken care of. The statement may need to be repeated several times until the person gets the sense or feeling of the meaning of the words.

Incontinence can be one of the straws that breaks a carer's back, especially when the person is urinating in all sorts of strange places, or hiding small parcels of faeces around the house. It's a bit discomfiting when these are handed with great gusto to an unsuspecting visitor or used for finger painting. It may well be that the person with dementia is unable to find the toilet, or does not recognise the toilet when they see it. Some people find that organising a regular toileting routine helps with this.

It may be that the person with dementia has reached the stage where the messages are not getting through to the brain that the bladder or bowel is full. Carers also need to be advised that incontinence can also be caused by a urinary tract infection or a bowel which is impacted. In other words, there can be numerous causes which need assessment before the person with dementia is labelled incontinent when it is really a medical or management problem.

Incontinence aids may be helpful at certain times. However, carers should be alerted to the fact that they can be shredded or flushed down the toilet.

Older women sometimes believe they are still menstruating, and families find pieces of rag rolled up and hidden in the most unusual places. I am always reminded of the story of a ninety-year-old woman who said she could not have a bath because it was that time of the month. No amount of coaxing could convince her otherwise.

Suggesting that workers provide carers with the type of information discussed assumes a knowledge base that workers may not have. If this is the case, information on the majority of these issues can be acquired.

Residential care

When assisting families to make decisions about residential care, I've always had the conviction that it is important that all possible avenues be explored with a view to keeping the person at home for as long as possible. Reassuring carers that they have done everything humanly possible to keep the person at home helps to ease some of their feelings of devastation and guilt. I am sure that even if carers know intellectually that they are not able to manage what's left of the person, emotionally it is a different story when they see the person ensconced in some type of residential care.

I believe that some of this agony could be spared if carers were given counselling and support at this time. I realise that, in the real world, workers have heavy work-loads and that it is easier to take over the caring role rather than share it with carers. A change in the workers' attitude from carers being of only nuisance value around the place, to involving them from the start in the life of the residential care facility, may help to eliminate difficulties at a later stage. Carers have all sorts of information on the person both from a historical and present-day point of view which could make the lot of the staff person easier. Collecting and providing this type of information gives the carer a task, and at the same time gives them an opportunity to walk down memory lane and to look at some of the life-time achievements of the person.

It may also give them an occasion to examine some of the not so good times and to come to accept them for what they were. Staff would, then, also have an understanding of who and what the person was before the onset of the dementia, and of some of the things the person had been involved with during their lifetime.

Visiting

I always encourage family members to visit. Telling them the person will not remember once they have gone is not helpful to them at a time when they are trying to come to terms with the fact that they have lost this person for ever. There is much evidence to suggest that people with dementia do realise at some level that people do belong to them, and sometimes register a flash of recognition of the visitor. Many a carer's story testifies to this.

Transition from home to residential care

It is my experience that, for the person with dementia, the settling-in period in residential care is much more protracted and complex than for residents who do not have problems with their short-term memory.

There are some fundamental reasons for this. The person will almost certainly not have consented to the move and if they are still able to speak will rightly ask the questions, 'Why am I here? What have I done wrong?' or will assert strongly, 'I am not sick and I was managing all right at home.'

These are all reasonable things for the person to say as they really believe them. When confronted with these questions, carers do not always know how to respond, because the person with dementia will continue to ask the same question over and over, raising yet again all the original doubts. When this is happening, I have found it is helpful to suggest that the carer do something practical for the person with dementia. If this procedure is repeated each time the carer visits, it may help to establish a different type of relationship at a time when the carer has a huge gap in their life to fill.

A second reason that the transition period from home to residential care is particularly trying for the person with dementia is that they are not able to learn anything new, while every moment is now a new experience for them. Imagine waking every day and wondering where you are, and who all these strange people might be, and why they are taking your clothes off.

We know that the intellectual function of the brain is damaged in the disease process. Therefore, people with dementia relate at a much more primitive, but not childish level. They understand and relate much more at a feeling level and can pick up intonation in voices, and even the unspoken word.

Touch is also very important. Rough handling will often get an aggressive response. The person then is labelled as being difficult, when, in fact, they are only responding to the way in which they are being treated. Imagine how carers feel when they are told that their usually reasonably amicable relative had to be sedated because they have been aggressive. They do, however, understand that staff also have to be protected, if it is explained to them in terms of the damage to the brain.

In all fairness to staff in residential care, they are often subjected to abuse. On a recent visit to a nursing home, I was introduced to a male resident with dementia who propositioned female staff around the clock.

There are two stories I would like to tell to illustrate many of these points. The first is the story of a family's reaction in the early stages of the disease, and the second a story where the only option appeared to be residential care for all concerned. Although the carers were dealing with the disease at either end of the spectrum, both experienced a crisis, a feeling of powerlessness, and the normal grief reaction. In both cases, the main carer had been labelled as difficult by many of the people who had come into contact with them.

The ageing elderly sister

One of the greatest examples of a carer being labelled difficult was in a family of two sisters and a brother all in their eighties. The eldest sister who was the main caregiver had a serious heart complaint; her brother had suffered a stroke and was paralysed down one side of his body; the youngest sister had been diagnosed as having moderate to severe dementia although she was physically fit.

This carer had coped for five years under these circumstances without any outside assistance. There were no other family members, and the carer had refused all offers of help from community services. Unfortunately, I was asked to intervene when the carer had a fall. I was asked to find residential care for all three at the same place, an impossible task. This story does not have a happy ending, as the three had to be separated and never lived together again.

There were several lessons in this for me: one was that the carer had waited until the situation was so desperate that the only resolution was for residential care to be found for all three. Some of the key factors were that the carer was a very proud woman, and had difficulty asking for help. She saw this as an admission of failure. She also had had trouble coming to terms with the fact that her sister had dementia, and really believed that her sister would get better even though she had been told to the contrary. Denial was a very strong element in this situation. It mitigated against a solution in the best interests of the carer, and perhaps, everyone else for that matter.

Marital dispute or dementia

In the second case, the person with dementia was in the very early stages of the disease and was a much younger married man. Nevertheless, the case still has a number of similarities in the way the carer handled the situation.

Mr L. had distinct personality changes and had changed from a caring affectionate man to a critical person who said all sorts of hurtful things about a family member who had died years before. He was, in fact, reliving much of what had happened in the past.

Mr L. did know that he had trouble with his memory but believed that the main source of this was marital problems and not dementia. He was still able to drive his car and would go out driving for hours

on end. Mrs L. was very hostile about her husband's behaviour
and this had affected their social life.

The situation reached a crisis point very early in the disease
process and we had to find respite care for Mr L. This was equally
difficult, as in the first case, because Mr L. was a younger man. A
respite place was found. This had a stabilising effect on Mr L., who
was relieved to be out of the house and away from his wife. The
break enabled Mrs L. to make some long-term plans through
counselling without the added stress of having to care for Mr L. at
home.

By way of comparison, in the first story it was the carer who had
been identified as being difficult, and was denying the fact that her
sister had dementia. In the second it was the person with dementia
who was not able to come to terms with his loss and was proving
to be very difficult. However, in both cases, the lack of appropriate
care at a time when it was needed was an issue. One wonders what
the outcome of the first case would have been if we had, in fact,
been able to offer the carer counselling and community services
which would have maintained them at home or, as an alternative,
residential care for all three.

Each of the sufferers in the stories had someone to care for them.
There are many thousands of people with dementia who do not in
fact have any family carers, who live alone and appear to have no
links in the community.

I had the opportunity in 1988 to set up a home-based program
for people with dementia in the inner eastern region of Melbourne.
I encountered a large number of informal carers who were, unbe-
known to each other, supporting at home people with dementia who
otherwise would have been in residential care.

Informal carer networks

Informal networks in local communities are not a new phenomenon
and have been in existence for centuries. However, the existence
of several of this type of network proved to be invaluable when I
was involved in setting up the community-based program men-

tioned earlier. It was established specifically for people with dementia.

The aim of the program was to discover what families and people with dementia needed to remain at home for as long as possible in order to delay the need for institutionalisation. In the early stages, there were many impediments to the setting up of the program.

Carers were amazed at being asked what it was they needed to assist them in their caring role. Local service providers believed that this new program would duplicate their existing services. Once the program was in operation, they conceded that it was not doing so. Their services were not able to meet the needs of people with dementia and their carers. They had so many rigid criteria for eligibility, and only had a limited range of services to offer which had been developed for people who were not experiencing short-term memory loss.

While the program was being developed, the workers actually went walking with the people with dementia. They discovered that they had an informal network of carers throughout their local communities who had, in fact, been caring for them for months and sometimes even years. The interesting thing about this network was that they were not known to each other, because the person with dementia could not articulate to the various members of the network that the other people were involved.

In most cases, the people with dementia lived alone and had no close family members. For them, this informal network of people played a significant role in keeping the person at home long after they would otherwise have been admitted to residential care.

During the course of developing a case plan for the people with dementia, the network people were brought together, either at the program office or at a convenient place in the community. The result was that the informal network of carers was educated about the disease, and assured that their efforts to care for the person had been beneficial.

One of the main features of the program which acted as a reassurance to the informal network that they were not operating in isolation, was the provision of a twenty-four-hour service via an emergency beeper which was carried by a staff person at all times.

The experience was that the network did not abuse the full-time nature of the service but only used it in an emergency. However, there was one elderly woman, an informal carer, who was so taken by this new piece of technology that she tested it on two occasions to make sure it worked. She was delighted to discover that the staff person responded within a short period of time.

We used the same model of bringing people together when there was disagreement in families as to who was doing what. Providing a forum for families to be exposed collectively to education about the disease and an opportunity to ask questions about particular behaviours cleared up several misunderstandings and re-established relationships which had been damaged as the result of a parent developing dementia.

My work with people with dementia and their carers has been a very rich and mixed experience. I am glad that I went to it with a fairly open mind. I do, indeed, realise I have learned a great deal about the tenacity of carers and the way in which people cope in the most difficult circumstances. I've learned a fair bit about myself as well.

Anne: Nursing my mom

Loving daughter — reluctant nurse

I was both resigned to, and distressed by my mother's illness, right from the beginning. As a nurse working in a small country hospital, I was no stranger to *senile dementia*, as it was still diagnosed in the late seventies. The familiar symptoms were unmistakable as they began to develop in my mother, even in the earliest stages. I tried to prepare my father and sister. But we were used to Mom forgetting things — we are a forgetful family. And the increase in visits to the toilet, well, we were used to that too and she *was* getting older, in her seventies now.

We didn't think of taking her to a doctor, not at first anyway. I knew there was nothing to stop the disease. Mom had been taking vitamin B and lecithin, and all the currently fashionable, hopeful cures for years, to no avail. Her diet was excellent, her health extremely good. It always had been and she has, still, extraordinary recuperative powers.

We look back to the year she turned seventy as the probable beginning. That year she had a vague viral thing that, for a few days, reduced her to a frail old woman. This was shocking to us as she was such a vital, active, intelligent and involved lady. At the time, she looked sixty, and no one would have believed she was eight years older than my father, a fact that has blessed us through the hard caring years.

Had Dad been the older one, he could never have maintained the exhausting physical and emotional commitment that caring for Mom was to demand.

She recovered quickly, as usual, but was never quite the same — something of the keenness and zest for life was gone and her mind seemed never quite so sharp again.

In my work, I was confused by my reluctance to nurse the older, dementing patients. I had loved the *oldies* in earlier years, yet now I experienced feelings I couldn't account for, or even bear to acknowledge quite often. There was impatience, anger and an inner anguish and pain that I quickly suppressed with shame. Nurses don't get emotionally involved, even with their mothers. It was years before it dawned on me that I was her daughter, not her nurse, and this terrified, hostile, alienated, deluded stranger was *my mother* whom I loved and was losing, had lost, somewhere back there.

Mom's illness was characterised by fear and depression, and all the aggression that went with it. We could never tell her that she had Alzheimer's disease. She feared it so greatly. She had helped nurse her own mother through dementia, and remembering her own pain and struggle, she had often told my sister and me to put her 'straight into a place if she ever went like Gran'. After Gran died, Mom filled her life with mentally stimulating hobbies and activities to ensure against the possibility.

One of the more poignant features as the disease progressed was seeing, one by one, all these skills slip back out of her routine — 'too hard on the eyes' or 'couldn't match the wool'. There was always some valid reason.

The painting saddened us most. Dad tried to encourage her by doing some himself, and gave her the perfect excuse: 'I never get a look in now. Dad's always using the paints.' A while later, painting helped Dad fill the gap when she was in care.

Remembering Gran, it was with strong feelings of *deja vu* that we began searching for spectacles and keys, cardigans, books and the little sharp knife, began answering the same questions over and over, began insisting that Mom write down arrangements, began asking to speak to Dad when we rang instead of leaving a message.

I called more often, on the way to and from work, after shopping. The grandchildren couldn't sleep at Gran's any more; she panicked at the responsibility. But my daughter, in her early teens, spent many happy hours with her, doing things and playing games. The children accepted the changes in her, easily at first, in their different ways, but they missed the special relationship they had all had with her, especially the girl and the youngest boy, only eight or nine when the problems began.

An alien world

The progress of the disease has been slow for Mom, twelve years now, and still a while to go. This meant that for several years my parents could continue their custom of spending the cooler months camping on the opal fields. In fact, Mom loved and was better in the casual, private freedom of the bush camp, without the pressure of civilisation. It wasn't until her beloved camp became an alien and frightening place for her that they finally stopped going.

Mom had loved to take long, solitary walks bird-watching. Eventually, her keen sense of direction failed her, and she began to lose her way in the featureless bush. This was a terrifying experience for both her and Dad. She felt trapped at the camp. Even at camp there were further difficulties. Using the heavy camp oven for cooking on the open fire, which had once been an exciting challenge, became a frustrating and confusing burden. The purchase of a *Porta-potty* didn't overcome the problems of night-time toilet trips.

For me, the earlier years were not so bad. Mom was still Mom and with allowances, we could share our news, play Scrabble, and go for walks. She felt in control of the visits. Dad would use the time to get on with his work about the place or to get away for a while.

It became less easy as Mom grew more confused and suspicious, and more afraid of being abandoned. This became an obsession with her. She began to dread Dad leaving, even to slip up to the shop for milk and a paper. When he needed to go away for a whole day, she would be convinced we would never see *him* again! Later, the fear became a conviction that someone was threatening her and

Dad was a kind friend, there to protect her. (Mom was a rigidly moral lady, but she had no qualms about sleeping in the same bed with him!)

Later again, Dad became the unknown aggressor, the assailant, there to 'steal Ken's things', and murder her. There were times when she would be tragically convinced he had struck her, others when she would furiously challenge and goad him to do so. Sometimes she struck him.

Had she been able to find the number, she would have driven the police crazy! She did ring the numbers she could find, friends and relatives; not mine so often though, because I was usually not *her* Anne. I, too, went from kind and helpful friend to a conniving home-wrecker or home-stealer, in the more confused times. All women became the 'other woman', including me and the gentle nun who came sometimes to play Scrabble with her!

I found this very difficult to adjust to, although I pretended to myself that it didn't matter. I sometimes caught myself arguing with Mom, urgently trying to 'make her see' that I was really her loving daughter. Only today can I admit with hindsight how deeply hurt I was by Mom's lack of recognition of me as a person, especially when she held up my more distant sister as a paragon of gentleness and love! Thank God, my sister and I could share this together and laugh about it with love and support for each other.

Domestic changes

As her skills and concentration slipped away Dad took over more of the household chores, leaving for her those she felt comfortable with — sweeping, washing the clothes and dishes and cooking the meals. I visited more often and for longer periods, trying to be there for some time each day, although this was not always possible.

Mom liked the familiar appliances, like the ancient, leaking, wringer washer and the old-fashioned toaster. Eventually my sister gave her an automatic toaster to save on burnt bread. There was no relief from the regular floods in the laundry, however, when Mom decided to wash without Dad knowing. Finally, Dad drilled holes in the floor to let the water out!

There were often visitors from near and far. The opal mining life had opened them to many friends and many buyers, and they called sometimes for meals, and, occasionally, for a bed. Mom was a good hostess, but problems multiplied.

First, there was the shopping. She would go in with a list of six things, and come out with a cart full of everything but. Later, she bought the same few things, day after day, and I would be sent home laden with milk, eggs and butter that they would never use. Ultimately, she was able to allow Dad to do the shopping and be grateful.

Then, there was the task of getting the meals! She was a good, simple cook, always with canisters full of homemade goodies. These went first. Bought biscuits and cookies were helped out by generous neighbours' offerings from time to time. The canisters remained full though, often with stale or even mouldy crumbs. I began regularly checking the containers.

Breakfast was easy — cereal and toast. Mom ate well, but not before she had tried to palm off half her meal to whoever sat beside her! Dad bought easy cuts of meat and they always had cooked vegetables for lunch because Mom could peel them. She began peeling them as soon as they finished the breakfast dishes. By nine-thirty they were ready to cook, or cooking if Dad turned his back! Many a day, lunch was ready by ten-thirty, sometimes with two lots of lunch simmering away in separate pots. Once, Dad found, hours after lunch, a complete roast meal sitting in the fry pan, cold and ruined.

Often he would ring in the morning to see if I could eat with them, there was so much food prepared. One Sunday, we called on the way home from church. I could see a nice lunch was almost ready and at the appropriate time too, so I bustled the children off before too long, wondering at Dad's odd expression. This was soon explained.

'Mom' said one of my four boys, 'that was their second lunch!'

But when visitors came, Mom panicked. So unless I could be there, Dad would explain and they would eat elsewhere, or bring a meal with them.

By tea-time, Mom was too tired and confused to help much. Dad made something simple like soup, or sometimes a neighbour would bring food in. Often I would leave tea ready, or bring something in from home.

Dad was unable to bring himself to use Home Help or Meals on Wheels. Mom continually maintained that she did *all* the house-work. *And* the garden! We knew there would be outrage if a stranger came in to do her house, or cook her meals. There *was* outrage if my sister or I were caught doing the hasty clean-ups we always tried to get away with. If Dad had to be away for a few days, she and I would move in and stay, and while one of us talked or played Scrabble with Mom, the other would feverishly attack the bath or the walls, or a messy cupboard.

Washing her favourite clothes was even more challenging. They had to be spirited away before she dressed in the morning and she was always highly offended. Sometimes, her frustration sent her slamming out the door in silent rage. At first, we thought she would be away down the road, but invariably, two minutes later, there she was, pottering among the weeds in her dearly-loved garden.

Changing roles

I found it very difficult changing roles with my parents. For Mom, I did the motherly household chores, but I also needed to make decisions for her, guide and direct her like a child, comfort her like a child. My nurse mask helped me to detach myself a lot, but sometimes, when Mom was especially fractious or cunning, the mask would slip and the strength of my feelings would frighten me — anger and resentment often, and then guilt.

I was also parenting Dad in some ways; being there for him, both as a physical support in caring and as an ear, someone to whom he felt safe telling his own feelings of anger and frustration and pain, and of his fears and loneliness.

At first he couldn't grasp the nature of the disease. He needed to read it in print before he could hear my explanations and begin to believe that, maybe, he wasn't going mad, or was in some way responsible for Mom's condition. He reached desperation point before he was able to talk about her, even with me, but once he began the floodgates were open and relief was immediate.

We soon began to highlight the humour, the absurd, and often our helpless laughter saved an otherwise unbearable situation. He still felt disloyal and critical though, wanting above all to maintain Mom's dignity.

He found it very hard later too, to stop giving Mom choices which she couldn't make, rather than simply telling her what they would do next. He wanted desperately to avoid conflict and have her calm and happy, a hopeless goal, and his struggle was very painful.

The waking nightmares

I think the most difficult thing for my father was the lack of sleep, because his continual exhaustion made it nearly impossible to think clearly. Even when I was there with Mom, he couldn't allow himself to have a nap so afraid was he to drop his guard.

Night-times were terrible. Mom became caught in a waking nightmare of delusion and hallucination. She was certain the house was peopled with unknown 'others' who must not be disturbed or who were in some way threatening. Sometimes she believed there were children in her care, and she couldn't find them. She sobbed over imaginary rejections, arguments, blows, hysterically sometimes.

As fast as she lay in her bed, she would be up again to the toilet for the tenth time. Dad counted over twenty visits one night. If she wasn't up for the toilet, she would have to check the spare beds, or she was on some vague mission she couldn't or wouldn't put into words.

Only once did she actually go out of house. There was a tricky lock on the door that she never mastered. She wasn't a serious wanderer; she was too frightened to go out of sight of the house.

We found it difficult to change the night behaviour because Mom reacts oddly to medications. We settled for a simple sedative, *Noctec*, which usually gave them from three to five hours sleep.

Every night Dad ran her bath and gave her the tablet. Then he directed her undressing and saw her into the water. While she bathed (though I'm sure she didn't wash in later years), he collected her array of night clothes, including thick bed socks and a woolly jacket. Mom felt the cold. Then, he handed them to her, one at a time. Any change in this routine usually meant the laid out clothes disappeared, not to be found for days!

Mom's capacity to hide things was extraordinary. Eventually she began to have an occasional trace of wetness on her underwear, not true incontinence, but enough to galvanise her into action. She began surreptitiously folding up little pieces of toilet paper, rag and tissues, and secreting them in handy places. After she was placed in care, I filled a big black bin with what I found about the house! Although I kept a supply of panty shields, she preferred the more familiar, old-fashioned rags.

Throughout these years I, like everyone, had my own family dramas to contend with. Perhaps the most traumatic of these was the sudden near-fatal illness of our third son, who was left brain-injured, with personality changes and an impaired short-term memory. By God's grace, and with a lot of work by many caring people, he became nearly well with the passing of time. At first though, he was much sicker than Mom. The three of us played countless games of Scrabble, he and she distractions for each other. As the months went by there came a day when I couldn't choose between their conditions. Then the balance tipped, as he improved and she slipped further away.

Going home

Mom passionately wanted to return to her and Dad's childhood home in the hills, and as she became sicker the desire increased. Conversely, Dad found it harder and harder to get her there. They were accustomed to taking frequent trips there. Mom would stay with her sister or a friend while Dad pursued his business. Dad would use a forthcoming trip as a distracting treat when problems arose. But she began to balk, and finally wouldn't go at all, meanwhile bewailing the injustice of being kept from the one place she wanted to be. Dad had prepared a flat he owned there for them to live in, so that, when she needed care, she could be placed in the excellent and familiar geriatric hospital there. For eighteen months she found excuses — wonderful, bizarre excuses — why they couldn't possibly go.

How slow we were to see our mistakes! We had forgotten that poor Mom couldn't even decide where the cups were. How could she plan what to take on a day trip, much less face the prospect of moving house? Having realised, Dad changed his approach. Over a few weeks he took car loads of belongings to the flat, while I stayed with Mom. Then, on the chosen day, he simply loaded her up and away they went. After they left, I filled my car with familiar, personal things, her pictures, small pieces of furniture, clothes, ornaments, favourite utensils, and followed.

When I arrived, Mom was standing on the verandah in her raincoat, bag in hand, about to brave the torrential rain. She wasn't staying *there*! Dad looked desperate. Five minutes later, her pictures on the wall, familiar things around her, she thought she was in her own home again.

I stayed five days with them, three sleeping there, then two sleeping at my aunt's, so that it became their home. We put labels on everything — drawers, cupboards, doors. Some of them she couldn't comprehend. When I left, everything was in running order, as simple as I could make it, and I was a nervous wreck. I didn't understand I was grieving. Mom had slipped, lost a lot of her drive, in that move.

Assessment

Mom had been assessed about eighteen months earlier, but it was not an accurate assessment. She was able to maintain her 'social face' until she was very ill and she performed beautifully for the geriatric assessment team. Dad was too shy to try and set the record straight. Other than that, the only medical attention she had was the occasional trip to the local doctor, whenever we could find an excuse. It was not easy because, as she would quickly tell you, she was never sick.

We also had a few visits to a psychiatrist. He was a friend of my uncle, who was a psychiatric nurse. The psychiatrist diagnosed Mom and saw her twice. After that, she was so outraged by the whole affair that Dad and I took the appointments in turn, while the other looked after Mom. This doctor prescribed *Melleril* for Mom, but her night dementia increased with it, so we returned to the security of *Noctec*.

At this stage, however, we arranged for another assessment, and this was a different matter. The 'social face' had tragically slipped and plans were promptly made for day care, and respite care in three weeks' time. Dad's exhaustion was plain to see, as were the problems he was having in the caring. Mom, amazingly, agreed to day care which had been beneath her contempt before, and loved it! My sister and I went about organising and naming her clothes and packing for the big day.

We anticipated any number of hassles. Instead Mom said, 'How nice to have two lovely girls who'd do all this for me!'

The decision to keep Mom in the hospital was unanimous, fast, and devastating to Dad. He had drained all his emotional reserves to let her go for three weeks. He couldn't accommodate permanent separation. *I* was flooded with relief.

Hospital care

The assessment ward was beautiful, light and airy, and full of plants. I knew Dad was at breaking point. He didn't see Mom for two weeks while she settled, and his grief was painful to watch.

I found the ward to which she was transferred much harder at first. Lovely staff! But the day room? Crowded, full of chairs, full of dependent elderly women. My first impression was one of gloom and lifelessness. This was my mother's worst fear realised. I put on my coping nurse mask quickly.

I rose to the occasion with professional aplomb, dealt with admission details, calmly reassured my family, discussed with the staff what personal things to bring in.

Under a grateful facade, I guiltily suppressed the sick knot in my stomach and the tears I longed to let go. 'Oh Mom! How could we leave you here?'

I talked down to her, impersonal and encouraging, trying to keep the edge of anger out of my voice — anger at my own helplessness to make things right.

It didn't take us too long to see the life and love that was really in that ward, where Mom still is, and we thank God that she can be there today.

It was three months before Mom settled. Then, abruptly, fear left her. It seemed as though she realised she no longer had to prove anything, to pretend. She could just *be*.

There, under supervision, medications were found that helped her sleep at night and she adapted to the routine.

Today, over three years later, she is very dependent, but still sits up in her chair daily and is very strong. She became noisy and disruptive for a time, and developed tardive dyskinesia (the spasmodic involuntary movements of mouth and tongue, arms and legs) as a side-effect of the medication. It seemed difficult to find just the right combination of drugs to suit her.

A year ago, she had a seizure and a fall which fractured her pelvis. It seemed like a disaster, but, because of the seizure, different medication could be tried, and the one she receives now has changed her in many positive ways. For the six weeks she was bed-ridden, she knew us again, by voice and face, by name. Those visits were so special to me. They were healing and full of love, love shared and spoken.

Separation

So great was my father's commitment to his role as carer that he found acceptance very hard. He couldn't separate his life from Mom's and for month after month his day revolved around the time he spent with her at the hospital. He grieved bitterly, isolating himself, unable to let go of his guilt at his perceived failure as a caring husband. Only gradually has he come to a point, during the last year, when he could take up his own life beyond the hospital, participating again in his old activities and pleasures without feeling he is abandoning Mom.

Today Mom loves to be cuddled and hugged, and reaches out her thin, wasted arms, turning her mouth up to be kissed among her murmurings. Her only problem at the moment is her eyes, painful, with inverted lower lids. In a few days, they are to be corrected surgically. She turned eighty-two last week. Dad and my aunt, Mom's sister, visit her most days; usually they feed her her lunch. I have further to travel; I try to visit at least every two weeks, more often if I can.

Sometimes, just for a moment, she knows that I'm there.

Joan: The key word is care

'Now we can all imagine Henk arriving in Heaven and asking, "Where are the tools and what is to be fixed?".'

These were the final words of the eulogy at the thanksgiving service for my husband. It had been a story of a friendly, fun-loving man who had happily used his creative talents to solve problems. The light-stand for the organ, the carved legs of the communion cabinet, and the silver christening bowl were souvenirs of his handiwork. Every minor crisis had been turned into a joke — like being trapped on the roof-top during a cyclone in Fiji. People were still smiling as they left the church to the joyous music of Purcell's Trumpet Voluntary. Acknowledging the words of sympathy, I too could smile. Most could understand that my feelings now were of relief rather than grief.

The shock of four years ago had caused a kaleidoscope of emotions, the worst of which was guilt. But that feeling was gone now. I felt only relief and gratitude that Henk's total loss of memory had made him quite unaware of his situation. He had not suffered, had not known of my agonies.

Now, knowledge of dementias is more widespread. Causes and cure are still being researched, but correct diagnosis is more frequent. I had blamed myself for not seeing the risk involved in the surgery to remove a slight blockage to the left carotid artery. Henk had not been considered a potential stroke victim. He had no problems with high blood pressure or being overweight; a cholesterol test had never been suggested. Slight angina had been diagnosed, so when the surgeon mentioned a three per cent risk we had not asked, 'What risk?' We had both assumed it meant heart failure and immediate death. In our early seventies, neither of us feared that. But Henk was a perfectionist. He wanted to be rid of the slight tremor in his right arm. Even that had been deemed the result of a severe attack of shingles following a car accident some years before.

Dramas and misleading clues

Now the last fourteen years of Henk's life seemed as a film. A series of dramas interpreted each time as a misleading clue. Extraordinary situations in different countries. A script-writer could not have made it more exciting.

It was August 1976 that he had chosen to retire one year early from his desk at the State Electricity Commission, to spend his leisure in travel, adventure and good works, he said. He would also indulge in his hobbies of painting, leadlighting and creating metal sculptures. But first, he would enjoy remedying the faults he had found in our newly built town-house. Disdaining the lift, he had climbed eleven storeys to work each day, and taught a weekly fitness class. After lunch, all envied him the ability to sleep for ten minutes in his chair, and wake up full of vitality. None doubted his bodily health and strength.

He chose my absence on a Saturday afternoon to replace a roof tile. On my return, I found him in bed.

'Think I fainted,' he said. 'But I lay flat a while before coming down. I had better put away the long ladder.'

I persuaded him to rest while I phoned our doctor. A locum came and could find nothing wrong. But an ECG on Monday would be wise. After a good night's sleep, Henk awoke as bright as usual. The ECG revealed nothing abnormal. Perhaps mild angina was the verdict. 'Carry some *Anginine* in case of another attack,' was the advice.

We had a holiday in Malaysia with no troubles, and touring Borneo gave only continued excitement. I could not believe that Henk had a health problem but the *Anginine* tablets were always with me. He did an oxywelding job on the second storey of our church hostel. When I learned about it later, my worry was that the ladder could have slipped, but he was always conscious of those risks.

Next summer we enrolled for a volunteer work-party to build a chicken-breeding house at a Mission School in Fiji. I could only wash dishes or clothes but Henk offered for electric work or plumbing. We passed a careful health check and I did mention Henk's fainting attack. 'Take some tablets with you,' said the doctor. But if anyone could have needed tablets it was me. Warned of the coming cyclone hours before, the whole party had taken refuge in the school-house — that is, all except Henk. Desperate to ensure the spouting on the very high chicken-house roof, Henk had failed to secure the ladder. It was blown away with the spouting, leaving Henk to survive by the power of his arms clasped around the strongest beam. The deluge that followed almost ripped his clothes off before native girls watching from a window saw his plight and brought a ladder. He laughed heartily at our fears and suffered no ill-effects.

A year later we flew to England and joined a tour to Cornwall. While I researched family history at Penzance, Henk booked a day trip to the Scilly Islands, departing by plane and due to arrive back at six o'clock on the evening ferry. I was waiting at the wharf but Henk was not with the party. A lady told how Henk had given first-aid at a street accident and then fainted. 'But he recovered quickly and will come on the eight o'clock helicopter,' she said. Back at the hotel, a phone call reported that a thickening fog was delaying all flights. I had a night of worry until he arrived at six in the morning, seemingly well but very tired.

Henk had established a workshop in the stable on an estate which had been left to our church. The old mansion was reopened as a child care center and there were many jobs of conversion and maintenance. Later, a nursing home would be built on part of the land, but the project would continue for years. Henk went there almost every day.

Our lives assumed a general pattern with an overseas or Australian trip each winter. There were never-ending volunteer jobs for Henk during each day, but in the evenings he could relax with a book or his favourite classical music, if there was not a class for painting or furniture polishing. And he wrote many letters to family and friends in Holland.

In 1980, we took a coach tour to Central Australia. Henk climbed Ayers Rock with ease, only commenting on his stiff arm and leg. 'It's obvious that you have a short left leg,' quipped a passenger. 'The right one has to work twice as fast.'

Next winter, we stayed a while in Holland before joining a small group of Dutch people in a bus to the Dolomites. Our base was an inn in the little Austrian village of Bad Mettendorf around which we could walk or take easy climbs. The climax was a funicular ride to a mountain peak and then, for still braver souls, a descent into an ice-cavern. Not brave enough even for the funicular I chose to walk alone in the forest and meet the carriage on its return to the station. But Henk was not there. With the guide, he had completed the icy descent and return, then walked out and collapsed, unconscious, and blue with cold. The guide said that this was not unusual. Henk had soon revived and would come on the next car. He did, and gratefully accepted hot tea with an *Anginine*. There was no doctor in the village, but Henk was easily persuaded to stay in bed for the remaining three days. When we left on the bus, he was back to normal, but I was very worried.

By the time we reached Australia, the event had become insignificant for Henk, but not for me. Our GP heard the story and made an appointment at the Neurology Department of our public hospital, where tests were made and medication prescribed.

The next holiday was to Western Australia, travelling in our own car. We investigated gold mines, got lost in the desert, dug ourselves out of a swamp. Henk could cope with every emergency, his only slight complaint being irritation on his right arm, hand or leg. 'Blast those shingles,' he would say.

We postponed the next trip to Holland in favour of seeing Queensland and the Barrier Reef, again by car. Having been years before on a coastal coach trip, we chose the inland roads, sometimes driving for hours without sign of life. Henk had to change a tire and replace a broken fan belt with a stocking, but luck was always with us — and we needed it, when we had to get a tow to Charters Towers. Henk still kept his six-monthly appointments at the Neurology Department, and took his medication.

We went by car to attend a Summer School at Bathurst in New South Wales. Diverted by flood waters, we had two days of constant driving. Recent surgery to my hand prevented me from helping. Henk started the painting course with his right arm in a sling and the brush held in his left hand.

The winter of 1984 was Henk's last visit to Holland, and I saw for the first time his 'fainting attack'. We had journeyed by train to the southern city of Dordrecht, to visit our alcoholic godson. The young man had tried every treatment without success, and was newly divorced. It was an emotional occasion, in the lounge of the small inn, but we were talking quietly when Henk suddenly grabbed his right arm and gasped out, 'I'm paralysed. It's dead.' He stiffened out in the chair and became unconscious. I screamed for an ambulance, but there was a doctor nearby and Henk was revived in a few minutes, and capable of talking. He was willing to go to hospital, but demanded the special Heart Hospital in Amsterdam, which he had known when he was a member of the police force in that city. There was an express train soon and, seeing that Henk could walk reasonably well, the doctor agreed.

We were at the Heart Hospital two hours later. The waiting room was full but, on hearing our story, the desk clerk pushed a button and Henk was whisked away on a trolley. Much later a doctor appeared. I told him that I could not understand medical terms in Dutch, but his English was good.

'There is no immediate urgency,' he said, 'but your husband does need treatment. As you are tourists here, I suggest that you see Dr Blank who advises visitors.'

Henk returned looking pale and worried. The appointment with Dr Blank was for the following week, but Henk phoned KLM. Seats were immediately available on the next plane to Melbourne.

Our GP and the neurologist were not interested in the Dutch written report, so the same tests were repeated. Cardio-vascular disease was diagnosed, but surgery was not imperative. Physiotherapy plus exercise could help. 'I can't live without my right arm,' begged Henk. He was long-listed for an operation.

We both had faith in that hospital, but a series of nurses' strikes erupted. Almost a year went by as four times the surgery date was postponed. Each time caused outbursts of frustration, but Henk carried on with his jobs and his painting class, sometimes using his left hand. One day he collected the car after service, but the mechanic said, 'There's nothing wrong with the accelerator, it must be your leg.' Henk admitted that his right leg had been feeling weak.

In November 1985 the date for surgery was once more cancelled. Henk's frustration was acute. A friend had had similar surgery at a large private hospital. Our GP agreed to a change of plan, and the new specialist put Henk in hospital for two days of tests. There was a blockage in the left carotid artery and surgery was appropriate. A date was set for 19 December. When I said goodnight to him on the previous evening, we were both full of confidence.

The operation scheduled for early afternoon was delayed until five o'clock. The surgeon phoned me two hours later: 'He came through it well.' I slept easily until woken by a trunk line call from the same man already at his holiday home.

'The hospital has notified me that your husband suffered a stroke during the night. He will be conscious, but probably a bit groggy.' I was surprised, but not too worried.

Would he ever know me again?

Shock, amazement, disbelief, anger. All these emotions surfaced when I saw Henk. A few days in hospital, he had thought, was a small price to pay for more power in his right arm. Now I doubted that he would ever leave the hospital.

'Yes, the surgery was successful,' I was told, 'but in the night he suffered a major stroke.' Frantically, I sought a reason. Never having had high blood pressure, he had no stroke potential — we had both believed that. And he had twice coped well with anaesthetics. In fact, the car accident had revealed him as a superman when he returned to work after six weeks. Extricated from the wreckage with fractured sternum, ribs and arm, plus thirty stitches in head and shoulder, he discounted warning of shock. 'I survived the bombing of Rotterdam,' he had laughed. But there was a periodic reminder of that accident in the recurring attacks of shingles.

Now, with him connected to various machines in Intensive Care, I wondered if he would ever know me again. His eyes followed me, but there was no recognition. I should not have agreed to the surgery. But would he have listened? Just occasionally he had said, 'Don't do my thinking for me.' Guilt triumphed over my other feelings. Daily I sat by his bed, watching for some sign, listening to encouraging words from the nurses, and concerned about the absence of the surgeon. 'A doctor comes every night,' they assured me. I demanded his name, but each day the name was different.

On Christmas Day, Henk began to recognise me with a smile. He was moved from Intensive Care. Then he noticed noise. Sounds attracted his attention. The squeaking locker door irritated him. 'It needs oiling,' I told a nurse, delighted by his interest. Next day he climbed out of bed, and wound up his back rest. Putting the sides down was easy. I was overjoyed by this progress, though still he had not spoken. 'Speech and memory is affected,' I was told, 'but therapy can do wonders.'

Four weeks passed before the surgeon returned from his vacation.

'Don't be impatient,' he said. 'There may be some loss of memory, but speech therapy will help, and physio will improve his right arm. Henk is now ready for rehabilitation. He will be almost back to normal in three months.'

'Good enough to drive a car?' I asked.

'Maybe even that,' was the answer.

The Rehabilitation Hospital was nearer to home. It took me only two bus rides, instead of three, and less walking. I found him in a four-bed ward, but tied to a chair. 'He walks so well,' the sister said, 'but with change of medication, he will soon settle down.'

And it did seem that he would. He had immediate rapport with the patient opposite. Percy was paralysed but could talk. Henk acknowledged him with a left-hand salute and a smile. In the opposite corner was Jim, a quadriplegic. There was no doubt of Henk's concern for him. The fourth man evoked no response at all.

Each morning I arrived at eleven and was greeted with a beaming smile.

'It's Joan,' I would say.

'It's Joan,' said Henk.

'I am his wife,' I said to Percy.

'I am his wife,' repeated Henk.

He repeated everything I said. That was a new worry. But there were other encouraging signs. With a spoon in his left hand, he could feed himself. When Percy called for a bed-pan, Henk would find a nurse and pull on her arm. If Jim dislodged a blanket, Henk would replace it. He could walk alone to the toilet in the passage.

The social worker gave me an interview. 'There has been difficulty finding the right tranquilliser,' she said, 'but he can soon begin therapy.'

I was delighted to learn that the woodwork teacher was from Holland. I sought out the man and excitedly told of Henk's carpentry skills. 'He can even use tools with his left hand,' I bragged. Observing group therapy, I knew that bingo would not interest Henk, but anything to grip his imagination would get results.

My elation did not last. After two weeks all therapy was discontinued. There would be a conference to discuss Henk's future. My stepdaughter was invited. The inference was that Henk could not be rehabilitated. I demanded another brain scan, immediately. By this time Henk was walking out of the ward, and being followed when he passed the nurses' station. Sometimes, he returned willingly, but occasionally he resisted, and then had to be tied into his chair. They would again change the medication.

At the conference, there was an unpromising report from each therapist. The Ward sister interjected, 'But he appears to know so much — surely a place in the Hostel.' A doctor produced the new scan. 'The grey areas are so extensive.' They gave me three months to find a Nursing Home. I knew now that my last vestiges of hope were gone.

The long-range plan

I don't know how I reached home that day. But I do remember sobbing for most of the night — and accusing myself over and over. Praying for a miracle, I knew there could be none. I would give him some new quality of life. Perhaps the therapists had not tried everything. I must experiment myself.

With H E N K printed in large letters on a sheet of paper, I put a pencil in his left hand and guided him to copy. But he made no move without aid. I drew each letter of the alphabet and he dutifully repeated A B C ... but he did not know one letter, nor recognise his own signature. We tried in Dutch with no difference. He crumpled the paper; it was just a game. But Dutch conversation did affect him. It brought tears and unhappiness though he understood nothing of the talk. The Dutch friends were asked to speak only in English.

One morning, Henk found his way to the car lot and discovered an unlocked vehicle. He was trying to start the engine when a nurse caught up with him, and it took two strong men to get him back to the ward.

On another day the hospital phoned that Henk was missing, perhaps making for home. He walked in soon after, having come six kilometres and crossed an eight-lane highway. A doctor and two male nurses arrived to find him enjoying a cup of tea and enthusiastic to demonstrate his complicated music equipment. He returned willingly to hospital carrying his own portable cassette player.

Meanwhile, I was investigating nursing homes. The one of my preference belonged to the church of which we were members — but there were only two male beds. He would have priority, but it could be a while. His name was listed at several other places.

It was time to consider my future, and I recalled our long-range plan to spend our last years in the residence run by our church. We had thought to live happily in an independent unit where Henk could pursue his handyman hobbies while I would quietly write. The difference now was that I would be alone in a single unit while Henk was a few blocks away in the nursing home. The prospect was acceptable. Before my lone trip to Europe the previous year, we had given each other power of attorney, so selling our jointly owned house would present no difficulty, and the sale was arranged; moving time was flexible. In April, a bed became available for Henk, and there was a vacant unit for me. We each moved on the same day. I saw Henk settled in and seeming to know the place and staff. My worries left me. Surely this was the will of God. I had my first good sleep for five months.

Peace was shattered on the next day when a former neighbour arrived with Henk. His wet and sandy shoes indicated a walk along the beach. From there he had taken a familiar route to our first home. And now, seated in his own favourite armchair, he was completely at ease. We called the new GP who had arranged Henk's transfer. The urgent problem was security. There was an immediate bed in a private psychiatric hospital in the next suburb. (We learned the cause only later. When a belligerent room-mate had threatened a nurse, Henk had restrained the man by a judo wristlock of considerable force. In the commotion, he walked out.)

The new place was perfect for Henk. He could climb the stairs, operate the lift, and wander at will. He was escorted for walks and seemed to understand that he must not go out alone. He wore a permanent smile and cheerfully waved goodbye each time I left. My appointment with the psychiatrist explained that Henk was responding well to a tranquilliser new on the market, which would control his periodic aggression. But he had no psychiatric affliction, so his stay must be limited.

Meanwhile, I had to adjust to a new style of living in a motel-type unit. With limited space, came decisions about suitable furniture and articles of necessity. The contents of five rooms had to be dispersed. Heirlooms were allotted to young members of the family; relics from Holland to my stepdaughter Anita. Selling our collected antiques caused heart wrenching decisions, but the money was needed. There was risk of Henk recognising our car. I got rid of it too. There was so much to do and so little time. Friends began to comment on my loss of weight. That brought a smile from me. 'Worry must be the easiest way to reduce.'

Friends. My husband had been my best friend, but there were others. At first, I had encouraged their visits and listened to their advice. All believed that Henk recognised them and understood their conversation. He did seem to nod or shake his head at the right moments. It could not be total loss of memory. It was useless to tell them that Henk was just as willing to kiss the hand of any nurse or kitchen maid. Few had experienced the care of a dementia patient. There was more understanding from the staff at my residence. The supervisor suggested a solution. Perhaps Henk could now be accepted into hostel care. There was a vacant room on the same floor as mine. Approval was given and Henk moved in.

The building was very familiar to Henk, and most residents had known him as a cheerful, friendly volunteer, willing to fit an extra shelf or cupboard. But next to his room was a concrete stairway to the kitchen quarters and boiler-room. An unexpected noise could provoke his curiosity during the night. A folding camp-bed enabled me to sleep there. Mine could be our day-room.

Sleeping well again, I rose at seven o'clock and made tea. Dutifully Henk would swallow his tablet after repeating 'Good morning, Henk.'

'No. It's "Good morning, Joan!"' I would say with emphasis.

And he would earnestly repeat, 'No. It's "Good morning, Joan."'

His speech was perfectly clear, but never of his own volition. He could manipulate the hot and cold taps of the shower, but needed assistance for drying and dressing. He tried to help me fold up my bed, and was eager for the porridge made in the kitchen. He went alone to the toilet, only coming to me for his belt to be fastened.

He watched my every movement with interest until it was time for a walk to the shops. Carrying the basket was his claimed privilege.

At noon, I took him to the top of the stairs to follow others to the dining room, where he found his seat with those needing a vitamised, easy to eat dinner. After that, he dozed a while, and was then anxious for a physio session or another brisk walk. We tried every available group therapy, but none held his interest. He preferred the variety of walks. We could go to the very end of the pier and watch the boats. There were many streets with colourful gardens to admire. We fed the birds in the park and saw children at play. He seemed to understand my chatter.

I joined the evening meal to butter bread or help cope with soup. Then we listened to music or watched television until he looked drowsy. Still afraid to leave him alone, I also retired early. This pattern changed little for the next six months, but I was becoming tired.

A book that I had written was published; an author's tour was planned. At first, I said no, but the GP said that a change would be good for us both. The psychiatric hospital agreed to accept Henk again, and he responded to the welcome. Leaving him, without a qualm, I enjoyed the tour. On the day of my return, it was planned to collect Henk the next day, but the supervisor interrupted my breakfast. 'Henk is just coming up the path,' she said. 'Did he know you were home?' I wondered about telepathy. 'He watched us go to Mass,' said a nurse who arrived soon after.

Our routine resumed. By this time, there had been a few more 'faints', now diagnosed as transient ischemic attacks, or mini-strokes. Usually recovery came within minutes, until one morning it was different. The shaking grew to violent spasms. The alarm bell brought the supervisor and we got Henk to the floor before he became unconscious. An ambulance took us both to the public hospital where he remained in a coma for some hours. I was questioned about epilepsy in his family, but it had never been mentioned. By evening, there was still no available bed, so the psychiatric hospital admitted him again.

When I visited, he could walk with me to the open gate, and then return to the front door, giving a wave before disappearing inside. There was never an attempt to follow me. A few weeks passed and then he went out alone. Probing my brain for possibilities, I mentioned his workshop at the Pennell estate. The shortest route was five kilometres, but he was there. Cheerfully, he was returned to our residence.

There were only minute dramas for the next six months, until Henk's tranquilliser became difficult to get. The manufacturer told of increased demand and shortage of the imported factor. Small quotas of tablets were obtained in other suburbs. Henk became sometimes aggressive. I took to carrying a couple of tablets in my purse.

Out walking one day, when I said, 'It's time to turn back,' he seized my arm with a strong grip and almost dragged me to the corner. Turning in the direction of our last home, I guessed his intention and tried to say calmly that we would visit our neighbours. Almost running to keep up with his stride, I prayed desperately for help, then sighted acquaintances in their garden. Answering my call, they gave a greeting and offered afternoon tea. In their kitchen, I crushed a tablet into Henk's cup and gave an explanation. Thankfully, we accepted a car ride home. These episodes of aggression became more frequent. And then came a threat of another kind — an urgent demand for sex.

Since sharing his hostel room at night, it had become the custom to wake Henk with his tea, and then accept the invitation to get into his bed. He would wrap his arms around me and doze off again. Then, just occasionally, his sexual instincts became aroused and, with a little stimulation from me, he could complete the act to his satisfaction. It seemed sensible to me to confine these occasions to Sundays when we could sleep in. And Henk seemed to accept my explanation until, one day in the other room, he suddenly pushed me to the floor and made clear his intentions. Hastily grabbing some cushions, I tried to co-operate, but he had become as an animal using brute force, until we both lay exhausted. Later I told the supervisor, who phoned the district geriatric center and, next day, there arrived a doctor and nurse to interview us separately. Reluctantly I showed the bruises on my breasts, told about Henk's gentle nature and explained his allergies. I felt there was little chance that the episode would be repeated. But I was secretly afraid. The decision was that Henk should spend a month in their psychiatric ward for observation. There would be a wait for a bed.

The medication became available again and our routine life resumed for some months. Then, as I was changing my shoes for an afternoon walk, Henk gestured his impatience and stormed out. When I reached the gate he was turning into the lane connected to a busy road. The supervisor was in her office. She directed me one way, and took the other by car. When she sighted Henk, he was going into a service station. As she watched from the doorway he began to operate the forklift, so she ran in and seized his arm. He was threatening with a karate chop to her neck when a mechanic appeared. Henk recognised the man, burst into a smile, shook hands with him, and then meekly followed to the car. Back at our residence, it was decided that Henk had become a risk. The psychiatric hospital readily accepted him once more.

After some weeks there came notice that an assessment team had classed Henk for special accommodation, and I was given a list of places. One was far away, but being especially recommended, I went there first. The owner was proud of this well-designed new building and showed the single suite available. I was impressed, and mentioned that a trained male nurse in Holland was entitled 'Brother.'

His reply stunned me, 'I wouldn't have a trained nurse in the place. I pick my women and train them myself.'

The only acceptable place was run by a fully trained sister and had an electrically operated security door. The residents looked well cared for and there was a homey atmosphere. I agreed to pay extra for a visiting nurse to shower Henk each day, and his transfer was effected. He immediately inspected the door and demonstrated his ability to reach the high bolt and turn off the alarm. Diplomatically the sister positioned a special chair and appointed him doorman. Next day he let me in and insisted that he stay by the door. It was his job. And I complied by fetching another chair. I had no notion that the sister ran two other such places and only visited weekly unless called.

For two months Henk continued happily to let visitors in and out until he had another transient ischemic attack and the sister directed that he be sent to the public hospital. Meanwhile the scenario changed. A melodrama began to unfold in my own life.

A lesson well needed

With some security in the knowledge that Henk appeared to be settled came a sudden feeling of freedom. A brisk walk to a local boutique appealed. Approaching the railway crossing my eyes noted the boom-gates but my feet still turned to the pedestrian crossing. The train missed me by a metre, and the horror lasted for hours. It was a lesson well needed. Care for my own health was now imperative.

Pondering the problem of exercise and relaxation, I thought of the new indoor pool close by. Swimming was my sport and I had taught it for years. There was no time to waste. Next day, in the ill-lit building, I saw first a children's pool. In the other pool, at one end, were three men talking with heads together as they kept afloat with gentle breast strokes. My training would never permit a dive in unknown water, but I guessed at two metres depth as I leapt up — and then down — crashing heavily on one foot. The men were patients for hydro-therapy in very shallow water.

Knowing my foot must be fractured, I hopped to the steps and dragged myself out.

Later in hospital, with a cage protecting my foot, and less pain, sanity prevailed. I phoned to enquire about Henk, and heard that he was happy. Then the focus moved to my own plight and pessimistic thoughts crept in. Pinned down for eight weeks could I control events that may happen? My stepdaughter, Anita, had a husband, four teenagers and a career — and she lived some distance away. Trust was in a younger friend who lived close by. Rona accepted the responsibility, and enduring power of attorney for me was given. Rona could visit Henk, and I asked other friends to do the same. With time now to meditate, I decided that my prayers were being answered. My confinement became a holiday. The role reversal was really a pleasant change until the next adversity.

Reports about Henk were good until the sister rang. She thought that he would like to hear my voice so she held the phone to his ear. Talking to him was harder than expected. Would he know my voice? He had not noticed a telephone for two years. Would he, childlike, break up the ear piece to seek the person inside? The sister told how he appeared satisfied and seemed not upset, but I began to worry.

Nine weeks had passed before my foot could touch the floor. Rest and therapy had improved my spine, so I could go home with crutches or a walker. Decision was made for the walker, and I used it on my visit to Henk. He kissed and hugged me, and made gestures of sympathy. Then he transferred his interest to the walker and performed a parody of my action. For a moment he seemed his old self, ever looking for something to lighten life. I was not too worried when I left. But I had no inkling of the crazy comedy of errors to follow.

At noon next day came a call from the hospital which had so recently discharged me, 'Your husband is in an ambulance at the door. There is no information but his name. What do we do?'

The driver knew only that he had been given a patient for the psychiatric hospital, which was obliged to refuse a stretcher case. The receptionist advised the nearest big private hospital. It was lucky that I was known there, so I begged time to unravel the mystery.

It transpired that Henk had suffered an early morning attack and had been sent to the public hospital which had his record. Recovery came quickly so they sent him back to the special accommodation, but now the sister was there and she decided not to accept him. Knowing that he had been in the Psychiatric Hospital, she phoned there, and was told that there was a bed for Henk. So thinking to save me from worry, she phoned Anita at her office and asked that she transfer her father by car. Not understanding the situation,

Anita decided an ambulance would be more convenient. After this explanation, Henk was moved in to occupy the bed I had so recently vacated.

Now came another period of peace. That private hospital had been good for me: I knew the staff and, best of all, that particular room was far from outside access. It was an answer to my prayers.

The financial situation

With time to think, I began to consider our financial situation. After the sale of the house our lawyer had advised putting half the proceeds into long-term investment. The balance paid the ongoing fees to our residence and left plenty to augment our age pensions. With fringe benefits, top hospital cover plus extras had seemed unnecessary, but we had paid it for years and, since Henk's illness, I was grateful for that. But now the bank balance was seriously depleted. Private hospital and specialists' bills had been far above top cover, and insurance could not be claimed for special accommodation. Some medications were not on the free list. But health was our priority and I could use the investment when needed. After all, saving for the rainy day had been our long-range policy.

Our doctor now asked for Henk to be reclassified, and it was felt that he should go to a nursing home as a Category 3 resident. A social worker would help find a nursing home. Hearing of my difficulty in walking, Jenny came in her car and we discussed the list. Some smaller homes did not admit men, a few she could not recommend. I marked those nearest, or that could be reached by public transport. She offered to pick me up next day.

Jenny had made a rough map showing all nursing homes within a ten-kilometre radius. And there were several beyond that distance that she could vouch for. She advised me to write down comments about each place.

That first day was a real eye-opener for me. Old private houses that had been converted or had wings added, had steps or staircases that I saw as a danger to Henk. For one such home beyond the boundary I would need a taxi.

'But the nursing care is excellent,' said Jenny. Newer buildings had wider passages but some had a sterile look. In one of those the director of nursing proudly showed the male dayroom with five men sitting in stately splendour. 'I like my gentlemen to wear collar and tie,' she stated.

By the end of the third day, I had a.collection of cards and prices, and my list with comments. Unfortunately Henk was male, and the waiting lists were long. Jenny explained the new government rules and the application that must be submitted to the district office. It was necessary to choose four nursing homes and indicate a priority. It took a couple of days to decide. I revisited some with Rona or Anita, and asked their opinions. Finally the form was filled in and posted. At Jenny's instigation, I joined the local carer's group for Alzheimer's Disease and Related Disorders.

Meanwhile, my foot was improving. The first walk with my walker to the milk bar had been slow and fearful. I had to use taxis to get to Henk. My right foot was now bigger than my left and adjustments to shoes were made.

When Henk had been a few weeks in hospital, the insurance company began to ask, 'When is he going to a nursing home?' So I telephoned those on my list. The first said, 'He will get the next bed, but it could be months.' The next two said he had been moved up to second place. The fourth told that Henk could have the next vacancy. That home was within walking distance, but had a grim facade. I hoped it would not be needed. After weeks of waiting the call came. It was from my lowest priority. I asked for thirty minutes to consider, and phoned my first choice where the director of nursing had impressed me. She asked what had been offered and, on hearing the name, said, 'Take it. The nursing care is excellent.'

The next phase

Next afternoon Henk was moved to the men's ward for three patients. He was given a bed by the window and there was an open door to a small garden. I asked about safety. The door could be closed but not locked. The paling fence was two metres high and the gate to the front garden had a security lock. The ward was at the rear, and there was a long passage to reach the front door. I was warned that settling in could take a few days, but they would watch him carefully. For the time being he was well tranquillised.

When I visited next day, Henk was plainly upset. He could not be interested in the magazines I brought him. Suddenly he got up from his chair, opened the door and went out. I followed, but did not call for help until he climbed on a cross-beam and grasped the top of the fence. Two nurses came quickly and added their weight to mine, but Henk had a firm grip. The whole fence came down. He was given an injection and tied to a chair. I was now told that he had already climbed the fence, crossed the adjacent vacant block, and was followed to the next property before consenting to return. He was good-humoured and seemed to see it as a joke, so the staff had not been too worried. Now the door had to be locked and the fence hurriedly rebuilt.

Within a few days, the restraining belt was removed, and it was obvious that Henk was content. Frank, in the next bed, was younger but could not walk. He offered his friendship, and they became mates. They both disliked the other man: 'Because he is bad-tempered and keeps us awake at night,' explained Frank.

A friend to both was the young chef as he brought their food with cheerful chatter, and visited sometimes to share his cigarettes with Frank. The laundry maid also smoked with Frank when she came in to fold sheets or replace clothes. Henk had quit smoking over thirty years ago, so I was concerned when he put out his hand for a cigarette and took a few puffs. Fortunately, it did not interest him.

The staff liked Henk and he loved them, especially the European nurse who sang German folksongs and brought tears to his eyes. She would then waltz him around the room to regain his happy mood. Most afternoons I would sit by his chair with my knitting, after absorbing Frank's report of what had happened since yesterday. Henk could hold the ball of wool on his knees, and unroll it when I gave a gentle tug. When I brought a large spool of yarn to wind into balls, he gave it his full attention.

A regular important job for Henk was to carry empty dishes to the kitchen after the midday meal. Holding each article with both hands, it took many trips. After some months his walking skill declined, but he still kept his job. He could kick off with his good leg, lean his weight over the cart, manoeuvre through the doorway, and ride the long passage to the kitchen. The staff applauded his efforts.

To my knowledge Henk only went out alone on one more occasion. He was recognised by a shopkeeper who, from his door, watched him approach the railway crossing. But Henk stopped, looked a while, and then turned back. He shook hands with the shopkeeper, walked on and turned the corner to the nursing home as a nurse came looking for him. Her reprimand was halted by his obvious happiness to be back. After this incident I began to feel that Henk had found his final home.

As the year passed Henk enjoyed every planned function. On Melbourne Cup Day he wore a top hat with dignity and lifted it to the ladies in their feather boas and flower-decked hats. Frank could not join the party in the dayroom so Henk returned to keep him company. They were mates.

Meanwhile, on the Pennell estate, our church nursing home was nearing completion. It was larger than the one it would replace, so there would be extra beds. Henk was entitled to one of them. Dr H., a long time friend, would be a patient there. He and his wife had visited Henk in the rehabilitation hospital over three years ago. Speaking of her husband's early dementia, his wife had said, 'Wouldn't it be wonderful if they eventually share a room in our new nursing home?' I agreed that there could be no better fate for them both.

When the building began a year before, I had visualised walking Henk from the new nursing home to see the children at play, and then to visit his workshop in the stable. It could be a dream about to come true. But would such a move be too traumatic for Henk? Our doctor helped to make the decision.

The official opening was postponed, and then fixed for 20 August. By coincidence, it was also Henk's seventy-eighth birthday. Attended by former clergy, and parishioners, past and present, it was a chance to renew old friendships and there was much talk of Henk. It seemed prophetic that his life should end here.

Two weeks later he was moved into a room with Dr H. who could still talk and was able to give Henk a welcome. The only trauma was for Frank who had been left behind.

The final chapter

Now began the final short chapter of Henk's life. I had thought that he would fight to the end, but there was a surprising climax.

Calmly he accepted that he could no longer walk and sadly, I had to agree that even a wheelchair ride to the workshop was not sensible. In the afternoons he reclined on a waterbed chair by a window wall, with a view of the garden. I sat by his side and played his classical cassettes: there was no doubt of his good hearing. He co-operated with every function, and had a smile for each person who passed, but he no longer laughed. He seemed to enjoy his spoonfed meals, but grew more thin and frail.

Taking the opportunity of a bus trip to the mountains, I bought a bunch of red tulips, thinking he could not fail to recognise his national emblem. But his response was totally unexpected. 'Smell the perfume,' I said, holding a single bloom to his nose and clasping his hand around the stem. He pushed the tulip into his mouth and began to chew.

At that moment came the chilling realisation that Henk was blind.

Our doctor thought it likely that Henk's sight had been slowly deteriorating, or that there could have been a slight stroke in the night. I believed now that Henk was longing for the end. His face had relaxed into a permanent slight smile. I had seen and heard the signs of death so, when it happened on an afternoon, I called the sister. Henk had reached the new decade. It was 2 January, 1990. We could only give thanks for the peace of his passing.

My over-riding emotion, now, was gratitude. Foremost for Henk's total loss of memory, and then for my contact with the Alzheimer's Society. And our doctor for the past four years had been the right one, a young GP who had kept abreast of progress. His advice, that multiple infarct dementia had been identified as a disease only in 1974, had finally extinguished my feelings of guilt. If there was a fault it was one of general ignorance. Genetic clues had been elusive; both parents and older siblings had died of vague illnesses in war-torn Amsterdam.

Henk was in the wrong place at the wrong time. His physical appearance, mental strength and unwillingness to admit a weakness, had set the scenario for a serial that did not serve him well.

I was grateful that I had made the right decision to sell the house and be rid of that responsibility. Coping with the immediate tasks was not too difficult.

Soon after our marriage thirty years ago, we had discussed our funeral preferences. Henk would be interred above his first wife, in the lawn cemetery. My ashes would be scattered there. We had agreed on private ceremonies and no flowers. From time to time we had talked about the publicised needs for organ research, and decided that our healthy kidneys would not help. Now I had a different opinion. Though none of my family had suffered a dementia, it was still a possibility for me. I would record my health history and will my body for research.

The Alzheimer's Society had taught me much in my two years of membership. It was social worker, Jenny, who had urged my attendance at the local carers group, and there I found the people who really understood my problems. Everyone cared for a person in some stage of dementia, be it Alzheimer's, Parkinson's or multi-infarct disease. Seated around a large table at the monthly meetings, each told of experiences. We learned from one another, gave helpful hints, and laughed at the funny anecdotes. In their own homes, or in every kind of accommodation, daughters cared for parents, and spouses for each other. There was even a single son whose mother had a colostomy in addition to Alzheimer's. He had the floor tiled so that he could walk through the house with a hose when she detached the bag. I would be ever grateful for the support of these new friends.

Although my husband has died, I still attend those group meetings, and act as a volunteer telephone advisor at the Alzheimer Society office. From their library, I borrowed the latest text books after finding that the public library had outdated information.

Recalling that Henk and I had chosen our church because of its caring congregation, I realise that 'care' is the key-word. The carer is just as important as the patient.

After correct diagnosis of a dementia, what is needed is information. Most patients can be helped to lead happy lives, and they seldom suffer pain. It is imperative for the carers to take care of themselves. Yes, the key word is 'CARE'.

Barbara: Looking for the cues...

My mother has Alzheimer's disease. This reality has changed my life dramatically over the last twenty years. When my mother first developed the signs of the disease, I sought assistance. To my great dismay, I found little. Because the professional workers did not seem to know or understand, I accepted, in 1983, a position on a steering committee to establish the Victorian branch of the Alzheimer Society.

This involvement has taken me down many thorny paths since 1983. The Society has grown and flourished at a rate beyond which any of us imagined.

My mother was placed in care some nine years ago. I have watched with horror and dismay the way in which she and other residents have been treated. I have talked with many hundreds of fellow-carers and participants in support groups. I have taken a professional position in co-ordinating a program providing community based care for people with dementia, particularly those living alone. I have worked with and taught many people who work in this field. Through all these experiences, what has struck me most is the difficulty so many people have in communicating effectively with someone with Alzheimer's disease and the frustration of the person with the dementia as a consequence.

I write from my observations both as a carer and a professional working in this area for the last seven years. Much of the agitation and distress suffered by people with dementia, their friends, and their carers, both paid and unpaid, could be relieved if the nature and process of communication was better understood.

I remember my mother standing on the beach excited by the sights, the sounds, the taste, the smell and the feel of the elements. She said, 'It is so awful. I won't remember that I have been here.'

Similarly, I remember the story of a woman being driven home after an enjoyable day out: 'It was a lovely day, friendly people and busy. I won't want to go next time because I will have forgotten.'

So many people become confused about the nature of the forgetfulness of the person with the disease. If we really listen to the person with dementia and understand some of their history, we can often understand the intent of the person trying to communicate.

I expected people with dementia to still be able to process basic information reasonably efficiently. I had to learn to understand their difficulties in this area and in finding the words to reflect their feelings. I had to understand what a thirty-second memory span really meant.

I learned that, to communicate well with people with dementia, we must recognise the fear and frustration that builds up when people's behaviour changes to become so out of character and so difficult to understand even for people who have known them for many years.

The workings of the brain are complex and still so little understood. So much of communication relies on the way in which information triggers off shared understandings of concepts, past experiences, likes and dislikes, positive and negative emotions. For the person with dementia, it is often difficult to bring together the different components of such an experience. The influence of the manner or style of the communication is more important than its content. For example, if staff in a residential care setting are anxious or frustrated about something, such agitation is likely to be communicated although it is not being expressed in words.

Understanding people with Alzheimer's disease

People with irreversible dementia seem to touch their heads a lot, hands tense, foreheads furrowed with worry.

Many say things like:

'It's all in here.'

'It's not in here.'

'It's all black in here.'

'There is nothing happening.'

'It's awful. I forget all the time.'

'Do you realise I've forgotten how to spell a few words. Shows how the brain has withered, doesn't it?'

'Did I tell you earlier that I was in hospital? Only nerves and misery! I think they thought I'd lost all my marbles. Maybe I have.'

'I asked did I still have a brain. They said 'yes'. So maybe I have, but I've no energy.'

For a long time, many people with Alzheimer's have a great deal of insight into their loss of memory, their muddlement, their making more and more errors, their inability to adequately do things that they have done with ease all their lives. The language they use to talk about their insight does not follow a rational thought sequence but expresses intent. One major lesson I've learned was about the need to look behind the words used at the intent of the communication and to use other cues to assess the correctness of my interpretation.

Alzheimer's disease prevents a person from realising the impact that their memory loss has on other people. Families, relatives, neighbours, friends, colleagues are bewildered by the changes beginning to occur in the behaviour and ability of this person. Often they are labelled difficult, lethargic, wilful, stubborn, disinterested, careless or clumsy. They may develop quick-witted ways of avoiding direct questions, respond with a question, change the subject or ignore the whole verbal interaction.

People don't need to be told they are losing their memory, they know it. They need to be assisted and supported in adjusting to their changing abilities in a way that encourages their self-esteem and confidence.

Historical context

It is critical to know the historical context and the life story of a person with dementia if we are to analyse, interpret and understand their changed behaviour and hence their attempts to communicate. If not, behaviour can often appear to be totally out of character and extraordinarily inappropriate. Such behaviour can attract responses that are fearful, frightening and humiliating. However, by understanding a person's background, past interests, habits and hobbies, I have found that I can, at least, try to put the behaviour in a context and find ways of dealing with it.

I will talk about Reg in order to link what seem to be vague meaningless actions and collections of words that apparently make no sense with the historical context of part of Reg's early life.

He had been in the dementia unit of a nursing home for some months. A tall, well-built man, still upright, strong and steady, he had a charming smile and a winning way about him. His wife and daughter travelled a long way to visit him and had cared for him at home until his wife's health and strength began to let her down. Reg was very restless in the late afternoon almost every day. Sometimes he was given extra sedation, and sometimes he was tied into a chair which also had a table screwed into the arms so he could not move. This made Reg very anxious and angry. When he was permitted to walk about, he began to push any movable chairs along until they were near the handrail on the wall. He collected cushions and left them on the chair backs. He collected the canvas ties that were used to tie people to chairs, and tied the chairs to the handrails.

One warm spring day, Reg was sitting between his wife and daughter in the sunshine, the gentle breeze lightly blowing his silver hair. He continually leaned over backwards and pulled leaves off the camellia bush behind, crunching them up in his hands and dropping the pieces on the ground. His wife said that he used to play the gum leaves very well as a young man when she first met him. His daughter went off around the street and brought back a range of leaves from different gum trees.

With a big grin, Reg placed them carefully in his lap and felt each leaf. He selected one and placed it between his two thumbs and began to blow. The thin squeaky noise of Waltzing Matilda could be made out from the sound.

His wife's eyes filled with tears. Reg said something like, 'I was a young'n out there in the red and those others told me about it and we did it and they went down and it was done all the time ...'

Big tears ran down his wife's cheeks as she said that she had not heard him talking like that for years. It seems that before he was twenty, he had worked on a station property in central Queensland and the Aboriginal stockmen had taught him to play the gum leaves.

His family agreed that his behaviour with the chairs in the corridor could well have been related to his long-term memory and the responsibility of tying up the horses each night and giving them their nosebags of feed. I have found that trying to make sense of seemingly uncharacteristic behaviours in terms of past history can help relatives and staff accept and try to manage differently some of the difficulties that arise.

I have to remind myself to think about a person who is eighty-five years old in 1990, as having been born in 1905 to parents who were twenty-five years old at that time and whose grandparents were fifty years old, born, that is, in 1865. The influences of language, social circumstance, historical context of the country in which they were reared will, in 1990, still be having an impact on this person. The knowledge is embedded deep in the long-term memory.

Take, for instance, the woman of ninety-two walking quite quickly along a corridor saying that she must go up the backyard. To a nurse of twenty-three in 1990, that might sound like confusion. However, those of us who lived in the 1920s and 1930s, and before, know that most lavatories were up the backyard.

Similarly, a woman of eighty-five would not now be looking for the washing machine into which to put the clothes. She would be looking for the washing board on which to scrub them.

I remember the story of a young male assistant who had a very dark rampant horse tattooed on his upper arm.

'How much did that cost you?' said the old woman who had been the secretary to a general manager of a large bank.

'How much do you think?' said the young man.

'Oh, I don't know because I have not brought my abacus with me,' was the quick reply.

Short-term memory loss

I have found that it's very important to understand short-term, mid-term and long-term memory when trying to communicate with people with dementia. I think it is also critical to try to understand how our thoughts, actions and our very being is tied so closely to our emotions. We all know that when we receive news of an event that gives us great joy, the powerful feelings of pleasure stay with us for a long time when we think of that event or person. Conversely, if we have been frightened, humiliated and frustrated, the awful, overwhelming, uncomfortable feelings remain with us until we can work through and reason our way out from the situation.

It seems to me that, for persons with dementia, it is possible for us to understand that they have lost that capacity to work new things through, and so are left with the 'awful' feelings which continue to be uncomfortable. I try to understand the ways in which behaviour changes as they try to deal with the feelings in an apparently inappropriate way.

For example, someone may have observed others walking down a passage and disappearing through a door at the end. They want to go out too. They stand by the door, but each time a person goes through they are pushed aside, until their feelings of frustration and fear of being trapped are so strong that they raise a walking stick threateningly at the next person who comes by.

It must be like a sort of nightmare where you can see what you want but can never get to it. And how many times do we have nightmares and are so glad to wake up and find ourselves in bed and not in that dreadful nightmarish position? We see people in this sort of situation quite often in nursing homes.

I have found that you need to accept that, in the here and now, a person with dementia could quite likely have a thirty-second memory span. If I accept this understanding, I am saved a lot of frustration and given the challenge of trying to avoid setting up situations that will not work. By breaking down the tasks into smaller sections and providing clear, slow instructions, I am able to communicate effectively.

For example, if I ask a person to go to the coat cupboard and get their coat out and put it on because we are going out shopping, I am setting that person up to fail at the task. I am also setting myself up to be very frustrated when perhaps not even the first part of the task is accomplished.

Constant failure to complete tasks which are no longer possible, then, affects self-esteem, confidence and competence. Because people with dementia often say things like 'What have I done now?' or 'Why are you looking at me like that?' we know that they are suffering feelings of insecurity about what they might have done that is in error, or what they might have left undone.

Abilities not incapacities

Not one of us would want to be caught shop-lifting, to have a store detective pounce and take us to the manager, talk and accuse and make an embarrassing fuss. Not one of us wants to be found to have wet or soiled our pants. People with dementia do do these things, which they would not do if they could possibly remember how they had always managed with competence.

People with Alzheimer's disease become unable to adapt to new ways, emotional climates and often new physical environments. This is especially difficult when the sufferer is a younger person and the spouse–carer finds that the balance of interaction in the marriage/partnership alters quite distinctly, that is, one has to do the adapting, compromising all the time while the sufferer becomes static and is sometimes called 'unco-operative'.

The old saying 'Out of sight out of mind' is so relevant in understanding some of the aspects of Alzheimer's disease. One who suffers from it loses the ability to initiate, to get things going or to follow through with sustained concentration. They cannot learn new things and they cannot hold new information in their heads for much more than thirty seconds at a time. Hence the importance of using cues in a variety of ways.

The strategy of using recent, large photos of people within her sphere of life, of objects to help cue into place an activity is indeed very effective in building or maintaining her confidence. For example, to show Sophie a photograph taken at the day center, with the piano (which is very important to her) and the co-ordinator, gives her an immediate understanding that that is where she is being invited to go now. She recognises that she has been there before and has good feelings about the time spent there. She cannot remember who the people are but she knows that they are fun to be with.

Creating cues through music is another useful aid to getting messages through. For example, Madge, aged eighty-eight, lived in a nursing home for several years. She was short, had a gravel voice and had played the piano in a music hall in Kalgoorlie before the First World War. Now Madge could not spontaneously start to play a tune; if she was escorted to the piano and made comfortable she would protest that she could not remember any songs. However, with the Women's Weekly upside down on the music stand and with the cue of someone singing, humming or whistling a melody, Madge would begin to play with gusto and could manage twenty songs one after the other without halting.

Similarly with Sophie, who had been a classical piano teacher; she had sold her piano twenty years before and had lost confidence. However, with her friend humming a nursery rhyme from her European folklore, Sophie began slowly and hesitatingly to play again. It is such a joy to see their pleasure at again trying old skills. The way the communication is made has to be right more than the actual content of the communication.

I know that it is so important to try not to ask questions that require the use of short-term memory. 'Did your daughter visit you today? Did you go shopping this morning?' This immediately puts a person in the down position because we know that a thirty-second memory span is about all someone with dementia can muster.

A person with dementia is quickly offended by a nurse arriving on the doorstep and suggesting that she/he has come to help with showering or changing clothes. This gives the message immediately that the person with Alzheimer's disease is not clean, is in need of help, is not quite good enough. In fact, this whole approach (which is still so common) sets up a confrontation, an angry feeling, a backing away from any help that might be offered.

So often in communication it is what is *not* said that gives the most powerful message. In talking with relatives of people with dementia in residential care, I hear them saying if only the staff listened to what their loved ones were trying to say so much frustration and aggression could be avoided. Aggression is often caused by the frustration of not being understood.

Photographs

In my own communications, I am finding photographs to be invaluable in enabling a person with memory loss to use their visual memory in a very positive way, so that dignity and self-esteem are preserved and enhanced and to support positive verbal communication.

Elsie, a widow of seventy-seven, has lived alone for ten years in a small unit on a busy road. She has no surviving children, and no relatives in Australia. Her friend has worried about Elsie being so socially isolated. The district nurse calls twice a week to organise the pills, and meals on wheels are provided for seven days. It was decided that day care would be worth trying and Elsie would have the opportunity to play the piano again. She had been a tertiary level teacher of the piano, but had to sell her grand piano twenty years ago for economic reasons. A first home visit of an hour established that Elsie would like to be called for and taken out to afternoon tea.

On the agreed date I went to her house, greeted her, introduced myself to her and asked if she would like to come with me to afternoon tea.

'But why should I come with you when I have never seen you before in my life?' she said.

I thought I could not say that I had already spent on hour with her and her friend in the house just a few days before. That would emphasise her loss of memory, create anxiety, humiliate her with her forgetfulness and be generally not conducive to forming a warm and trusting relationship. I rummaged around in my head to find a way of indicating that we had met before and that I was a safe person to go with. I then made a remark about the elegant paintings that Angela was doing at her painting classes.

'Oh, you know Angela?' she said.

'Yes, and I have seen some of her beautiful work.'

We talked some more of Angela and I suggested that it might be fun to phone her.

'Would you telephone?' she asked.

I did and told Angela that I had been visiting Elsie for some time and, yes, we were still at Elsie's unit. Angela understood immediately that I was having some difficulty and said she would like to speak with Elsie. They talked for a short time and Elsie put down the phone, collected her handbag and umbrella, checked all the doors and out we went into the sunlight and were on our way to the center.

The next week, a similar performance.

'But why should I come with you when I have never seen you before in my life?'

Again, it took about thirty minutes of my time before we were in the car.

At the center, I asked Elsie if I could take her photograph with Jean, the co-ordinator. Elsie was really enjoying her time at the center each week, but, of course, had no recall of events. I took a photo of them both with the piano in the background between them.

The following week I returned to collect her to go the center, greeted her and before she could begin with 'But why should I come

with you ...?', showed her the photo and said, 'The pictures have
come out so well.'

Elsie looked closely and said with a wide smile, 'Oh, yes, I have
been there before.'

'Well, would you like to have afternoon tea there today?'

She collected her handbag and umbrella, checked the doors, and
we were in the car within ten minutes.

The photographs worked each week. When I was away and
another member of staff went to collect Elsie, she took with her a
photo of me and a photo taken at the center with the piano. It
worked and Elsie went off confidently without saying, 'But why
should I go with you ....?' Now she does not need the photos as
cues. She is able to recognise us each time and has confidence.

Communicating with a person who has had Alzheimer's disease
diagnosed means different things to different people. For people
in a family who have known a person for thirty, forty or fifty years,
and who know something of the historical context in which this
person grew up, there is already a large knowledge base to use.
With the help of new information about dementia, a comfortable
understanding can be maintained for years even when the dementia
is quite advanced.

Another example. A man and his wife were standing by the
bedside of his mother (there were no chairs in the room). She had,
that day, had a severe stroke and was unconscious. The man held
his mother's hand. A staff member came into the room and
suggested that he did not need to stay as his mother did not know
him or know that he was there.

I was tending another person in the room and asked him, 'Are
you "my son, Bill, the jeweller"?' He turned his sad face towards
me and indicated that indeed he was.

I told him what a joy his mother had been in that ward and how
she told people with such pride about 'my son, Bill, the jeweller'
and how he married such 'a wonderful woman whom anyone would
want for a daughter.' We talked about staff not understanding the
finer points of communication with people with Alzheimer's disease and with those who are unconscious.

I suggested that his mother could be aware at a deeper level of her being that he was there. He said simply, 'Yes, I know, I can feel it in her hands'. His mother died peacefully that night.

We use all our senses all the time in making a communication with another person. We use gesticulations, some people talk more with their hands than with their mouths. We use words, our eyes, our whole bodies when we lean towards a person, or when we fold arms and lean back in a distancing way. We give a lot of messages by smiling or not smiling, by turning towards the speaker or turning away. Touch is one of our greatest ways to convey a message, holding hands and walking along together, taking someone by the wrist and pulling that person along. How we touch a person when we help them into a car, out of a chair, with a meal, with personal care; all our acts of touching give a feeling message to the receiver of our touch.

I know from my experience that people with Alzheimer's disease know that they are losing the ability to do things that they have done well in the past, they know that they are losing the capacity to remember how to do things that they have always been able to do.

This is indicated by statements such as:

'Do you mind me being a silly old woman?'

'Why have I got all these words and I can't find the right ones?'

'You must think I am mad?'

'Why can't I remember things? It is so awful!'

'I can't ever go to the bank again, I don't know why they were cross.'

Their communication to us at times is one of anxiety and panic.

'Who will tell me what I can do?'

I imagine that having such memory losses as we know develop with Alzheimer's must be like a nightmare from which there is no escape. The only avenue of communication that is left is through behaviour or by means of body language which can strongly indicate feelings. I think one of the most valuable lessons that I have learnt is to communicate through feelings which provide a secure emotional climate.

None of us likes sarcasm if it is at our expense. None of us likes people to be talking about our situation in front of us and without our involvement. None of us enjoys being organised and pushed around faster than we can personally manage and not one of us likes to feel that we do not have control over our own lives. So it is for a person with Alzheimer's disease.

I am convinced that we, as carers, need to learn a lot more about how our body language conveys information to a person whose feelings are their main source for interpreting what is happening around them. We have to learn more about using sight, sound and touch as cues to help a person with Alzheimer's disease understand what we mean.

If we add an understanding of how a lot of behaviour that is labelled 'aggressive' is really a response to fear, fright or frustration, I think we will come close to communicating with the people for whom we care.

But, most of all, we have to understand the nature and style of the dementing process itself if we are to make our communication more positive and supporting for the person with dementia. They know that there is 'something wrong with my head' and because of the disease process are quite unable to adjust.

Beth: Alzheimer's—
my companion of twenty years

My mother

Alzheimer's disease has been a companion of mine for over twenty years.

When my mother died about four years ago at ninety-two, she had run the whole gamut of the effects of this devastating disease. We had had to watch helplessly as the person we knew and loved gradually changed into a stranger who was devoid of personality and who required full-time nursing care.

She was a tall handsome woman at sixty-five, who had only a sprinkling of grey hair through her chestnut braids. She was in command of her domain and then Alzheimer's disease began to change her personality, and with time, transform her into a terribly frail little person who hardly made an impression on her bed linen, and had a gaunt, haunted, frightened expression in her eyes.

About six months before she died, it was decided that she should be X-rayed to see if there was any cause for the repeated urinary tract infections she was suffering. This entailed a frightening trip by ambulance from the nursing home to the hospital and back, and an X-ray that was all a waste of time and effort, because this demented person could not urinate on cue.

The urologist rang to inform us he was now going to put my mother in hospital to stretch the neck of her urethra, under anaesthetic. I challenged the decision on the grounds that, given her dementia, an anaesthetic would make her far more confused than she was already. I suspected that the procedure could be done with acupuncture.

He was horrified that I should question him and his method of solving the problem, and went ahead with it anyway. After that our mother couldn't recognise my sister and me. She was frightened of the dark abyss that she mentally lived in. For the last few months of her life, day and night, whenever she was left alone, she continually called out 'HELP'. Later, the word changed to 'HOME' and this made us feel even more helpless about her condition.

My sister did most of the running around that was required for our mother in the last few years of her life. She had elected to live in a special accommodation house of her choice after she had had a hip replacement operation. While she was in hospital, our father had caught the serious flu of that year and had died. The shock of Dad's death and all the trauma that goes with anaesthetics and operations sent her many steps down the road of dementia.

Dad had been her backstop, and she knew she couldn't manage without him and also, she had no desire to live with my family or my sister's. She understood the problems that were caused by three generations living together, as her own father had lived with us for the last few years of his life.

My husband—the early stages

I had little spare time at that stage, with problems of my own at home. My husband had started doing odd things, arguing about nothing, and becoming hysterical when small things went wrong. He didn't appear able to make rational decisions and was keeping more and more to himself.

He used to be very fussy about his appearance, but by that time he always had an excuse for not having time to have his hair cut. He was wearing jumpers with the elbows out. He decided that he only needed to have a shower every second day, and then he would always argue that he had had a shower yesterday. He wouldn't change his underwear and socks, and insisted that dirty or clean, they had to be out under his pillow at night. This, of course, was harking back to the cold days in the UK and also the times when the air raid sirens would go off during the war, and you would have to grab what clothes you could and head for the shelters.

I didn't have time to work out the source of his problem as I was working four days a week, trying to keep some equilibrium at home with our son, with rules about homework and school and sport. This was very difficult, as every rule was sabotaged by my husband shouting at me in front of the boy, and telling me that I was too hard on him.

My husband seemed to hate his boss, blaming everything that went wrong on him or some other employee. I couldn't understand his attitude, as he had been a kind man, with a pleasant sense of humour, with never a bad word to say about anyone. He was a perfectionist at anything he attempted, and so knowledgeable about every sport and sportsman that anyone wished to talk about, that I couldn't believe that this argumentative person was the man I had married. I even had to stop him reprimanding our son, as he had lost control a couple of times and hit him about the head.

And now my fears were coming true: he was not coping at home, and he was not coping at work either.

He worked in sales and as a storeman with a firm who sold and serviced motor mowers and chain saws. He was failing to answer the phone, was making errors on invoices, and would not use the new electronic cash register because he knew that if he made a mistake it would ring a bell, which would inform everybody of this.

He didn't want anyone to know he couldn't do things correctly any more. He would forget what day it was, where he had put a tool he had been using a minute ago, and the name of the customers he had been serving for ten years. He would even get mixed up about a circle of friends with whom we had been socialising for twenty years.

How hard it must have been for a man of fifty-two to admit to himself, or anyone else, that he was having such difficulties getting the day-to-day things right. No wonder he didn't answer the phone, no wonder he went out into the garage when the front doorbell rang, or didn't open a letter that was addressed to him. All of these things would have required a decision, or maybe talk about something he had forgotten.

At about this time, he was forced to retire from work, sick, and because the pressure was off and he didn't have to try anymore, he relaxed and cut himself off from the world of reality. He went into a huge black hole, and it took the medical professionals and me six months to get him back to anything like normality and pride in himself as a person.

My husband was too early with his illness. Ten years ago, no-one in Australia had heard of Dr Alzheimer, and his disease. No-one dared suggest that working in an atmosphere where carbon monoxide fumes were produced from the exhaust of motor mowers and chain saws, could affect a person's system or perhaps cause chemical changes which could alter brain functions and do damage to brain cells.

The local GP was sympathetic, the neurologist didn't have a clue what was wrong, and, referring to my husband, asked me, 'When did he stop thinking?' The psychiatrist thought I was a bossy woman, who never gave her husband a chance to initiate anything, because I had, of necessity, taken over all the household management.

Because I was not satisfied with the answers the doctors were giving me about what was actually wrong with my husband, I went into the area of homeopathic medicine. The homeopathic and naturopathic professionals and those who believed in alternative medicines could not agree that a person who appeared to be suffering the effects of some sort of toxification, should be prescribed anti-depressants. They said these appeared to be making him more confused and more ill.

Unfortunately for my husband, because of his low tolerance for some prescribed medication, and his own blood chemistry, he has been over-medicated and has had very bad reactions to drugs prescribed by traditional doctors at least three times over the last ten years of his illness. These reactions caused further liver problems, headaches and terrible skin rashes. One particular medicine had such a dramatic effect on him that he hit two nurses and had to be restrained until I convinced a doctor at the hospital that possibly he was allergic to the medication he was on. Once he was taken off this, he reverted to his old quiet self and could go back to his special accommodation house.

I challenged the traditional doctors about their diagnoses as to whether my husband was just depressed; had Alzheimer's disease; was suffering a bad reaction to their prescribed medication; had some other form of dementia; or was 'just malingering and had wasted five years of his life', as one physician had told me. I also challenged some of the things the doctors said, and I became very upset when I had to describe what I thought was wrong with my husband, and frustrated with the opinions they gave at other times. This made me unpopular with the medical profession, I was to them an unqualified person who was challenging their learned decisions.

Nonetheless, I still had to look after this person who was growing more and more difficult to manage on a day-to-day basis. He was not capable of doing anything constructive. He couldn't understand even slightly complicated instructions, and would become hysterical if the job was too difficult for him.

The psychiatrist he was attending was convinced that if my husband could perhaps have a small gardening round to do each week, it would give him an interest and encourage him to be his old self again. With the money from the insurance on our family car, which had been written off along with another vehicle due to an error in my husband's judgement, I went out and bought a truck so that he had a suitable vehicle for his mowing business.

Unfortunately, my husband had no idea of making money from the gardening. He used to spend anything he made on cigarettes and Kentucky fried chicken lunches, even though I had packed a lunch for him. I also had to pay the expenses for the truck to do the round and the motor mower's service, and the tools that were forgotten and lost on the round. There was the added worry that he should not have been driving a car. His ability to make quick decisions and also his judgement of distance were not good.

My refusal to renew his driver's licence when it expired caused a great amount of ill feeling, but three doctors had already told him he should not be driving. He knew then he could no longer drive legitimately and in spite of fiery words and desk thumping, it saved me much anxiety in the long run.

I had to learn to keep calm, never to raise my voice, never to lead with a question like 'Why did you do that?' because no matter how quietly I asked, or what emphasis I put on any of the words, it was always seen as an accusation. I had to convince our son that our lives would be far more peaceful if he never argued with his father, and appeared never to challenge his instructions. This made life quieter, but it didn't make it easier.

I am sure that we were never made to keep our emotions under control to that degree. The pressure generated began to affect my health and our son's ability to concentrate on his schooling. In addition, having a father whose illness no-one quite understood did not make him all that anxious to bring his school-mates home.

Having been prone to allergic reactions, I found that now my migraine and asthma were becoming much worse. My arthritis appeared to be progressing faster than it should, and my stomach nerves and general health were suffering. I was really living on the edge, constantly tired, with great difficulty in sleeping. I was trying desperately to take my husband to anyone whom I thought could help him to regain his health and to be the person he once was.

The battle begins

I was still working four days a week, managing the house and bills, learning about Social Security benefits, filling in forms for all manner of things that I had never had to bother about before, and trying to claim compensation for injuries received when someone wrote off my car from behind a year or so before my husband left work.

I had to convince Social Security that a man of fifty-two should be on sickness benefits, to convince the bank that since the personal loan was in my husband's name, their insurance had to pay it off, and to convince the insurance company my husband would never go back to work, and therefore they should pay up his superannuation. This all took about eighteen months.

I also tried to win a Workers' Compensation case, because I considered my husband had suffered brain damage in his workplace, due to the carbon-monoxide fumes. In 1984, three doctors were saying he had a toxic dementia. The other twelve doctors and specialists were calling it anything from organic brain dysfunction to depression to Alzheimer's disease — anything that wasn't going to open a can of worms in the Workers' Compensation arena. I had no idea when I started the compensation claim how involved and wearing such an exercise would be. Between seeing our own and their specialists, we averaged a visit to at least one of them each week for the four years it took for the case to be taken to court.

The attorney, who was supposed to be on our side, casually advised: 'You won't win. Take the money they are offering for medical expenses and give up.'

What compensation do you get for a damaged brain?

I was devastated by the no-care, no-help attitude of the Workers' Compensation company who were supposed to be supporting our cause. Our odds of winning in court were nil. I was too exhausted to fight back. My husband knew he was being cheated, but was simply unable to back me up in public. Our son was too young to stand up in the courts.

The doctors and the specialists showed a negative attitude to my husband's condition when confronted with having to testify in court on our behalf. These days, doctors will talk about toxic dementia; at that time they wouldn't. Whenever I have spoken publicly since about Alzheimer's disease, toxic dementia and incorrect medications, there have been statements from the audience about similar experiences. I have also heard many stories about people becoming ill or confused after working in the petrochemical industry for long periods.

One doctor who spoke after me at a seminar agreed that he had seen a number of Alzheimer's patients who had been farmers and had handled chemicals all their lives. There were the nurses in the audiences who nodded their heads when I spoke of over-medication and the effects of drugs on dementia sufferers. One swallow does not make a spring, but...

Investigating alternative medicines was an expensive exercise, but the reactions of my husband to normal medication raised questions about the dubious benefits of anti-depressants and the like. Anti-depressants and high-powered medications are less important to dementia sufferers than love, understanding, a friendly safe environment, and plenty of space to allow for their restless wanderings.

The first psychiatrist had insisted that we go on expensive holidays, 'because that will make him feel better,' and when that didn't work, suggested that I take anti-depressant pills so that I could cope with my husband's problem. I finally convinced myself that life wasn't meant to be that hard. I had my husband admitted to a private psychiatric hospital to get another opinion, and also so that I could get some rest from the merry-go-round I had been riding for too long.

From there, things changed; more opinions were sought. Alzheimer's disease, or possibly a toxic dementia, was diagnosed. I was advised more constructively how to face the future, and what I may expect to happen as time passed. I was told in no uncertain terms by one of my favourite doctors that I had not caused the illness. This altered my thinking, as it is easy to blame oneself. Did I give him the wrong food? Did I use the wrong cookware? Have I been too hard to live with, making him depressed and starting off this vicious cycle?

I finally began to take in all this well-aimed advice. Up till then I had been pushing myself relentlessly to discover the miracle cure, or at least to give the problem its correct name. I also realised that, if I became really ill, our home environment, such as it was, would fall apart. There would be no-one who could attend to all the practical details that had arisen because of my husband's illness.

At the time, I found that family and friends listened and gave advice, but offered little if any physical help. My husband's family all live in England; my family were still adjusting to my mother's death; our son was not mature enough to understand all of the problems. Friends were standing back from this terrible mysterious mental illness. I became so distressed when I talked about it or the problems I was having with the medical profession that it was much easier to keep out of ear shot, at a distance. I felt I was pretty much alone.

However, professional people at out local community health center were excellent, as were the other carers in the local carers group. Staff from the Alzheimer Society became my backstop.

After my husband had been admitted several times to hospitals and numerous tests, X-rays, CT scans, and blood tests, I decided that I had to keep working to pay the bills, and to maintain my sanity. I also decided that I was not born to be a full-time nurse, and I would only resent being tied to the responsibility of a dementing person who had lost his ability to comprehend the sacrifice necessary for one person to give up their life to care for another twenty-four hours a day. This is what caring for a dementia patient amounts to.

I had seen my mother slowly go into a decline, and the problems and heartbreak that that had caused, and I felt I couldn't go through all that again, first hand.

I put my husband into a special accommodation house, carefully selected. There were no suitable private special accommodation houses in our area. This was to have repercussions in the future. At that stage my husband was unco-operative, although he could go out walking for hours at a time and not get lost. I chose the most suitable place I could find at the time. The woman in charge was a registered nurse. The patients ate good food. The place was clean and had a large rambling garden.

That place was eventually sold, but they were happy to take my husband with them to another special accommodation house that they ran. However, when they took their business a good way out of town, I decided a change was needed. I knew the proprietor of a place specifically developed for dementia sufferers, the only one I encountered that was asking questions about what really were their needs.

He was accepted there and was able to stay in that safe environment, away from the world of decisions and telephones and challenges, for three years, until his condition deteriorated and he began to have seizures and had suffered two or three minor strokes.

The seizures took him to the emergency room of the local hospital on a couple of occasions. I tried to convince the resident doctor that he could not expect sensible answers to his questions as my husband had Alzheimer's disease, or a toxic dementia. I told him that, if he examined him, he must realise that my husband was not as sensitive to pain as a normal, well person.

I give credit to many of the doctors and medical professional people I met along the way for their knowledge, compassion, and understanding, but some I remember most for their arrogance in dealing with a patient and a carer, who were both frightened of what the future held.

A major decision—and more battles

I asked our son, who was having a great deal of trouble facing up to the realities of life at the time, what we should do about his Dad when he came to be discharged after a long spell in hospital. We discussed whether it would be better to bring him home, or place him in a home suitable to his mental capacity. We would resolve to do everything else we could for him, but, at the same time, get on with our own lives. It was a major decision. I felt more strongly than our son that putting him into care was the right thing to do, but in a short time he came to realise that it was the best thing for all of us.

My family were sympathetic and understanding of my decision. Some of our friends were with us all the way; others were uncertain, but accepted that I knew what I was doing. Still others thought that I was the worst in the world, but were not really willing to walk in my shoes.

One particularly good friend was able to look at things in a more objective way and he convinced me that I could give much more to many more people if I pursued the course I eventually took. On the other hand, I asked an old friend of my husband, of twenty-five years standing, if he would go to visit him in the special accommodation house. I thought it would be good if my husband saw an old familiar face from his soccer days. He went to see him all right, but then I received a quiet, but abusive phone call, asking me why I had put his friend in that dreadful place, with all those sick old people? I explained a bit about the sickness, but he never went near the place again. He never asks now of his old friend.

I sent my husband on a trip back to his family in the UK, while he was still able to travel, and was fairly aware of his surroundings. I felt it would be the last time he would see any of his relatives, and he enjoyed the six weeks he spent travelling from one family to the other, and seeing old familiar faces.

Unfortunately, some of them thought I was exaggerating about his condition — because we all know how well an Alzheimer's patient can keep up the image for a certain length of time and fool even the experts. When they decided to take him off the medication I had sent with him and which had kept him in reasonable health for four years — anti-depressants, many vitamins and B12 injections—I wrote a strongly worded letter of objection and explanation. Immediately they received this, they booked their brother on the first flight they could find heading to Melbourne.

In my husband's luggage was a letter written by the eldest brother-in-law, and telling me on behalf of the family, that I was a terrible person, a hypochondriac who was trying to poison their brother with all that medication, and who was trying to palm him off and shrug off my responsibility as a wife. I received another such abusive letter when I wrote and told the sisters that I had put their brother in care.

Their actions and lack of empathy had a devastating effect on me and also on my husband as he knew how much I had really tried to help him during his illness. I felt more alone than ever, but also that I was not prepared to face the illness alone any more. I wanted help, and I went out and found it.

In 1988, my husband was having seizures and had had two minor strokes, and so was generally beyond the care of the special accommodation house. He was still a very active walker and was out on the road, getting lost. He was put into a psychiatric hospital from which he couldn't walk away. They kept him in his pyjamas, so it was obvious he shouldn't be out of doors.

I was going on holiday, and felt he was in the wrong environment, with young disturbed patients, so I searched the southern and eastern suburbs, and found only one special accommodation house which would take active male patients. It had a high fence around a large garden. It sounded ideal, and the proprietor convinced me that I could go on holiday and not worry at all about the patient. 'The patient' had escaped by the time I was ready to leave home the next morning, but was found again before I left Tullamarine.

By the time I returned, he had escaped another three times, once overnight, and his medication had been trebled. He was walking around in a complete daze, and had lost about five pounds in weight. I was forced to admit him to that house because he could no longer be looked after at the old place. The psychogeriatric hospital would not accept him on family relief because he was only sixty-two, and they claimed that he didn't reside in their 'catchment area'. He had lived in the area for twenty-five years and had moved out to his special accommodation house only because there had been none suitable in our area at that time.

With help, the issue was forced, and he was allowed to live in the local cluster housing complex for about five months, until he became incontinent and got beyond their realm of care. In the first few weeks of being received at the cluster housing, he had to be admitted to a private psychiatric hospital to have his medication sorted out, because he was having blackouts every morning. These stemmed from the medication that some doctor had introduced some months before and which the people at the special accommodation house had tripled during his short stay there.

Again, because he was only sixty-two and still walking strongly, he could not be admitted to the local psychogeriatric hospital. He had to go to the under sixty-fives ward at a public psychiatric hospital on the other side of the city. He was too active to go into a nursing home.

He was well looked after there, but it is thirty-five kilometres to the hospital and as my husband was having seizures, the staff would call me to come quickly, as they thought he may die.

I appealed again to the local psychogeriatric hospital to have him transferred back to our area. When I got nowhere, I wrote to the Office of Psychiatric Services, and also to the Department of Community Services and Health in Canberra. A bed miraculously became available at the psychogeriatric hospital.

My husband is deteriorating further. About the only thing he can do for himself now is feed himself. The rest is left to nature, and all the doctors and staff required to look after him. The hospital is now talking about a nursing home when a bed in the right one becomes vacant.

Despite lots of consideration, my husband has been moved nine times in the past eighteen months, mainly because he was not sixty-five, and also because he was too physically fit for most of the places that are supposed to cater for dementia patients. I wonder if anyone realises how many clothes a dementia sufferer loses each time he or she is moved from one care situation to the next? Things are left in the laundry system and are never found again, so you have to buy new clothes with each move.

Does anyone realise how hard it is for a confused person to learn a new environment? When is the system going to look at these patients as people, not pawns that have to be moved from one situation to another when they progress from one phase of this devastating illness to the next?

The Future

When my husband had been in care for a short while, my lawyer advised me that, since there was no likelihood of his ever returning home, I could now consider myself to be legally separated from him, and if I chose, I could apply for a legal separation, and again, if I chose, could apply for a divorce after one year from that date. At the time this seemed to be all just words, something I would think about tomorrow.

But then one day, an old friend from the past appeared on the scene. He had difficulties of his own, and together we talked about them and gradually worked out our problems together.

It was marvellous to have someone to talk to who didn't turn everything you said into an argument — someone who could talk on the same level. We had a tremendous number of things in common, things that we enjoyed doing together. I had found a shoulder I could lean on.

I couldn't help my husband any more than I was doing. He was being well looked after in an environment that was suited to his needs and mental condition, and so I set legal proceedings in motion, and obtained my divorce. I made a financial settlement for my husband, so that he would have sufficient income, plus pension, for his needs for the rest of his life.

Since that time, I have remarried my old friend from the past. By the time we decided to marry, relatives, friends and professional acquaintances who had stuck by us through all the difficult times were delighted about our marriage announcement. These people all felt, without reservation, that we deserved another chance for happiness.

The ones who couldn't accept the news had drifted away anyway.

Although my circumstances have now changed, I still think that I should keep my ex-husband's well-being in mind. I visit him at least once a week, and always make sure he has enough clothes and other necessities. Now, I am told he has to go on to a nursing home, when a bed is available. That will require him to adapt to another environment, and another set of labels will have to be sewn on to more new clothes.

He has forgotten that I have divorced him, and I never talk about my new husband to him. I talk about our son, and those members of his family I still write to in England, as well as family here.

I am not sure now whether he understands all or anything that I say, but he smiles when I talk to him, and tries to tell me things, and I answer him as if I understand.

What more can one do for a dementia sufferer?

Bert: My wife, Joyce

Definitions and diagnoses

When I agreed to contribute to this collection of experiences of those caring for a sufferer of Alzheimer's disease, one of the questions I was asked was: 'How and when did you first start to be aware that there was a problem?'

I think this question should be restated: 'How and when did you first stop being *unaware* that there was a problem?' Because of the very slow deterioration in any single activity that goes with Alzheimer's, an awareness of any problem is *always* in hindsight. Looking back, say, one year, it is quite easy to detect the gradual changes that have taken place.

Once one is aware that some particular change has occurred, one also becomes quite aware of the extent of one's *unawareness* at the beginning. I always tried to compensate for these minute changes as they occurred, and it was this that initially and inadvertently started off the cover-up period, for both the sufferer and the carer.

This attitude has in the past been nurtured by the older doctors, simply by their reluctance to say the word, dementia. An American writer I like very much makes an attempt to show that the word, dementia, does not mean crazy, by reminding us that we older people learned our English sixty-odd years ago. My own dictionary is fifty years old. Bearing in mind that this is what we learned, let's look at what it says:

Dementia: Insanity characterized by the gradual weakening of the faculties.

Insanity: Unsoundness of mind; madness, *lunacy.*

Lunacy: Originally an intermittent form of insanity
              supposed to vary in intensity with the phases
              of the moon.'

No wonder there was a great reluctance of any knowledgeable person to say or even think of the word, dementia. No wonder many older doctors say 'Just a little bit of senility', or, in my case: 'She's too young to show these signs of senility.'

Perhaps it was this attitude throughout the ages that led to the absolute ignorance of Alzheimer's disease prior to 1985. It was certainly what prevented most carers of Alzheimer's disease sufferers from having any chance in the initial stages of even beginning to think about what may be wrong.

I find myself wondering what would have happened if Alzheimer's disease had been called 'progressive forgetfulness' leading to 'acute forgetfulness'? Wouldn't we have understood a lot sooner? I think so.

I cared for Joyce for six years before I accidentally found out what was really wrong with her. Once I had first-hand experience I was immediately able to recall other people I knew who could have had, or did have dementia, possibly Alzheimer's disease.

In 1931, as a young girl, my wife's sister visited Wells Asylum to see her mother's sister, her aunt, who had been certified. In those days, if you showed signs of insanity you were liable to be legally certified as insane.

In 1935, my father's friend's wife was found wandering near a railway line. Was she going to commit suicide? She was forty-seven-years-old. Certified and put in an asylum. It was very quiet. No-one ever knew what went wrong.

In 1953, when my father retired at sixty-five, he became very forgetful. My mother always called him Oodenead which is Somerset slang for Wooden Head. In 1964, one year after we emigrated to Australia, he died after being three weeks in a nursing home. He had lived on his own for two years after my mother died from a stroke. He was incapable. I now believe she also was a carer. No-one said what was wrong.

In 1986, my sister's children wrote to say that my sister had never answered any letters because she couldn't write. She had been the Matron of Southmead Hospital, Bristol. Other family wrote to tell me how stupid she had become. When they went to visit, she knelt on the carpet in front of the fire and never spoke a word. My brother-in-law cared for her until he was eighty-four. She's now in a nursing home. No-one said what was wrong. Dementia or Alzheimer's disease was never mentioned. She is now seventy-three and has deteriorated over twelve years according to the mail I received.

So, all of these people were sixty-five or very much younger at the beginning of their problems. Ripe before their time, precocious.

How rare is this problem? Methinks, not very rare at all. I think the medical profession works, or used to work, on the basis that ignorance is bliss. Believe me, a carer must understand to be able to accept. Must accept to be able to cope.

Joyce — the beginnings

In 1980, on a Saturday afternoon, Joyce complained of feeling queer in the head, a tingling sensation in her arm. She was fifty-three.

The doctor at the emergency room took her blood pressure, and the nurse did an ECG. As a result of this, tablets were prescribed. After a very gradual build-up of the drugs, Joyce's blood pressure kept fluctuating and different kinds of tablets were tried. She felt unwell, hazy and not in control, so spent several weeks resting. During this period, I took over the running of the house as well as serving in the small general store we owned. We had a fifteen-year-old daughter living at home and attending high school at that time.

Joyce slowly improved just as if she'd had a very mild stroke, and gradually took back most of the jobs she normally did, including serving in the shop when the occasion demanded, although the exception was the cooking of the evening meal which I retained, as it happened, forever.

I realise now that things she saw that needed doing she did one hundred per cent correctly. Things she couldn't see weren't done. This included knowing when to prepare a meal, when to start cooking the various vegies and meat, and when to turn it out and remove it from the stove. So it was that I did the cooking, but did not realise that Joyce's recent memory was now being affected. At half-past four Joyce took over in the shop and I started preparing the evening meal. At six the shop closed. Meal ready. Problem solved.

We spent a lot of time together in the shop. There were always newspapers and magazines to sort out, to write names on for the regulars, shelves to dust or to stack, stock to price. Either of us would serve and we were both able to tot up in our minds the total cost of two or three items.

On pension days, and at certain other times, some customers came with a list. We would write the prices down on paper and add them together. Joyce began to have difficulty in adding lists of about twenty items. Over approximately six months, the number of items she could total gradually diminished, and four items was the best she could manage. Eventually, she had to write down even two items to total them.

I thought this was due to stress brought about by high blood pressure which had reduced her power of concentration.

I bought a calculator. Joyce had a problem with this when the total answer ended in zero, because the calculator would cancel it. This is a one-in-ten possibility (eg: .33 + .47 = .8). This confused Joyce, who could not see that this was eighty cents. I was not at that time aware that this was the reason.

I decided we would not use the decimal point. In those days, most items were less than a dollar, so in any total the last two figures were the cents and the preceding figures were the dollars, and most importantly, the calculator no longer cancelled out any zero at the end of a total.

This worked very well for some months. Problem solved? No! One day I came back from the wholesalers, which was a weekly task, and found Joyce trying to charge a customer about fifty dollars

too much. He added it up for her and expressed his concern to me.
Perhaps she multiplied instead of adding? What her fingers did her
brain passed as correct?

Then I had a stroke and was in hospital for a couple of weeks.
Fortunately, this coincided with holidays, and our daughter helped
Joyce full-time with no problems at all. Joyce was still able to add
up two or three items on paper. Our daughter would check and also
took responsibility for anything in excess of that.

We sold the store and bought an old house on a large block just
outside of Maryborough. This was September 1982. Prior to this
we had been interviewed for naturalisation. This was granted on 1
September 1982, but it was four and a half months later before the
ceremony was performed. We returned to the Shire of Avoca
where we had to swear the oath of allegiance. Joyce was able to do
this in front of a crowd which included three members of parlia-
ment. Outside and in company, Joyce was normal and no outside
observer could have picked anything wrong at this time.

A couple of months later, Joyce began to develop a slight
difficulty in communicating. She had to think harder about what
to say in answering a question. This made her noticeably hesitant.
So, in the beginnings of this problem, there was no actual word loss.
Simply, the retrieval of words became more difficult.

To add to the complications, I had a heart attack, and spent a
week or so in intensive care. I was diagnosed as super-hyperten-
sive, and put on an invalid pension.

Joyce began to lose the ability to remember certain kinds of
words. Nouns seemed to be the main difficulty. We were at this
time both going to doctors. Because I needed help during my own
recovery, an occasional arm to lean on, someone to be with during
the frequent dizzy spells I was experiencing, I made our doctors'
appointments together. This meant that what Joyce seemed unable
to say or complete, I very surreptitiously filled in. I was very adept
at this, and I was trying to protect her from a condition for which I
presumed she was being treated. The medication list had grown
considerably for both of us.

While we were in the store, all of our food requirements were there for the taking. No need to go down the street. No lists for us. Now it was different. If she looked in the larder and saw items more than half-used, they would go on the list. However, anything we had used up and for which we had discarded the packets wasn't replaced. Roast dinner ready, no gravy. Washing up, no detergents. I began to help Joyce make up our list of requirements.

'Oh, what a tangled web we weave...'

Having now realised that something else was going wrong, the next time we went to the doctor's, I sent Joyce in on her own. I did this because I reasoned that she would probably behave quite differently. She had very much come to rely on me.

This resulted in tears in the comforting arms of the doctor, and an immediate appointment to a specialist. The doctor called me in and said it seemed like symptoms of senility, but at fifty-six she was much too young for that.

The specialist read the inevitable letter from the doctor, the contents of which we were totally unaware of. He arranged the interview so that I sat in a chair near a window, facing his desk. He was able to see me simply by raising his eyes. Joyce sat facing him close to the desk, with her back towards me.

'Right!' says he. 'I am going to give you four numbers to remember: nine, two, five, eight.'

'Repeat these to me!'

'Good and again!'

'Say them once more.'

'Excellent! In a minute or so while we are talking, I am going to ask you to repeat these numbers, so just once more say them now.'

'Good!'

He asked her various questions about past and present. I was unaware of their significance. However, if she hesitated, he looked at me in a manner that was almost imperceptible, and I either shook my head or nodded in acquiescence.

He asked her to repeat the numbers.

'Nine, two, seven, eight,' she said.

Not by a flicker of an eyebrow did he indicate that this was incorrect, and neither did she ask. By the same token, I never even discussed this interview with her.

'Oh, what a tangled web we weave
When first we practice to deceive.'

To me this was intended as a demonstration of the person I first met in 1941 losing, in two or three minutes, a part of herself. Neither of us was the same afterwards: we no longer felt quite as one. Feelings of deceit festered inside me until, some three years down the track, I had learned so much more about dementia. Only then could I begin to accept what had happened.

The specialist arranged for a brain scan, and also gave us another appointment to talk about the result. The good news was that there was no tumour or any other suspicious features about the results. We would have to look elsewhere for the problem.

Joyce had a red dye X-ray and an overnight stay in hospital to recover. The specialist arranged to meet me at Joyce's hospital bedside. The news was that her arteries to the brain were almost blocked. On one side only a tiny hole was left. A major stroke was imminent. A surgeon and the specialist decided to keep her in and operate. The first operation took place two days later. A by-pass to the brain, remove artery or cut open, clean out, replace and suture. Remove by-pass. Two weeks recovery and then a repeat on the other side. Four weeks in hospital and then home for recovery.

This was an extremely traumatic experience for me, especially waiting for the first operation to be completed. The nurse said that Joyce was going to surgery at one o'clock. 'Don't ring before five.' It is said that time is constant. What a lot of rubbish. That four hours took over a week to pass by.

We revisited the surgeon on three occasions, and then had three appointments over a period of nine months, to the specialist. At the last appointment, I said that she still had the tendency to forget names.

'What is this?' he said, holding it up.

'A pen,' said she.

'And this?' he said pointing at his wrist.

'A watch,' she said.

'She's not too-ooo bad,' says he.

'Do they ever get better?' I ask.

'Some do!' was the answer. But it was to be otherwise with Joyce.

During 1985 a number of activities began to show the early signs of deterioration.

We hardly ever used our phone, except to ring Joyce's oldest sister in England about four times a year. Most of our calls were incoming. For a person with dementia, the phone presents a problem because they can only listen to the caller, whereas in normal face-to-face conversation they are able to use a few visual aids.

It was noticeable that the conversation was gradually becoming one-sided. Joyce would answer, 'Oh yes!'

'Really?'

'No!'

'I'm not sure.'

'OK!'

'I do.'

It was clear that she was not really participating in the conversation. When people asked for me they would say they were having difficulty in getting through to Joyce.

Eventually she would pick up the phone when it rang and say 'I'll get Bert'. There was no longer an attempt to answer. If I didn't come quickly, she would just hang up. She was unable to say who called. She would get angry when I complained. 'Supposing it was urgent?' This kind of altercation was slowly to increase.

I decided to move the phone to the top of a small cupboard directly behind her armchair. The armchair faced the TV. When I went to the garden I would remove the handset from the phone. If someone called while I was out they would get the busy signal, and could call back if it was really important. Today, when the phone rings, Joyce takes no notice at all. She is no longer aware of its purpose.

It was a year since the operations. Occasionally, she seemed much better than usual. But surely if she were going to get better she should have shown some sort of overall improvement by now?

Our youngest daughter retreated to her room. She seemed to think that I was to blame for the emotional tension which was now creeping relentlessly into our home. 'Family problems due only to lack of understanding.'

Joyce's misplacing things became a common occurrence. She thought someone was moving these things on purpose. More trauma. This problem worsened because once she found something, she would deliberately hide it, so that only she knew where it was and then of course would forget all about it.

Another new trait: she would spend money from her handbag, forget she had done so, and then think it had been stolen. I spent many hours over the next year searching for things that were hidden, forgotten, and lost.

Our daughter ran away, with a man of course. She did call up and tell me. However, I've always believed the problem at home was the root cause. She returned with a husband many months later, but just for a two-day visit. Joyce had spent day after day on the veranda, looking for the white station wagon to return.

It would be an understatement to say that our daughter's actions disappointed me. Had I failed as a father? Regardless of my feelings, I am always reminded, as a practising Christian, of my boss's instruction: 'Forgive us our sins as we forgive those who sin against us'. And, of course, I forgave her.

Joyce also frequently realised that something was wrong, and her frustration and anger led her to the wandering off into the bush. Our home is surrounded on three sides by forested bushland. There are tracks along which we had walked many hundreds of kilometres together, but always together. The wandering became a daily occurrence. One second she was here, the next gone. I used to go looking for her, but usually the wrong way, and there was always the danger that she would return while I was searching in the wrong place.

In a strange way, her dementia was a blessing in disguise. After some time, she would forget that she was running away and her mind would simply revert to having a normal walk. She was not lost as the area was very familiar to her. She would return with no idea that anything was wrong. The initial wanderings were of about one to one and a half hours duration, but this slowly decreased in time, because she began to forget her original anger and frustration much more quickly. Eventually she reached a stage where she would go out of the back door, walk up the path, reach the edge of the forest, immediately forget what she was doing, and walk back into the house all in about thirty seconds.

Revelation

I began to feel lonely and wanted some outside contact. I decided to do the Community Information Workers course. Joyce attended the classes with me, although, of course, she was unable to participate. After completing the course, and doing three months probationary period, I became an accredited member of the Citizens Advice Bureau.

It was here in the pamphlet section, during 1986, that I came across a now familiar red and blue pamphlet called 'Dementia'. I sat down and read it. I realised that Joyce had all of these symptoms and some that were not mentioned. For a while, I had that deep sinking feeling, a large weight in the bottom of my stomach. Alone in that interview room, I began to gain an understanding, and more importantly, an acceptance.

Next trip to the doctor, I told him that I now knew for certain that Joyce had Alzheimer's disease. He agreed.

I had now been on my own with Joyce for about a year. By the end of 1986, I had become an eighty-five per cent carer. Joyce could wash, make-up, shower and dress herself, but everything else in the house was now my responsibility. She could still help with many things, but only under constant instruction and supervision. During 1986, continual deterioration of activities had become apparent, especially reading, writing, speaking and communication. Hobbies had also become affected.

I realised the enormity of the task ahead and contacted our middle daughter for help. She was a single mom who had been battling on her own for a few years, bringing up our grandson. She came home to help me. We bought a van which we stripped and redesigned for two people. She retained her independence, yet was just outside and able to give me some occasional respite.

While we were renovating the van, our daughter and grandson lived with Joyce and me in the house. Because our daughter managed to get a full-time job almost immediately, the van renovation took about nine months.

Problem-shooting

At that time, I didn't use any of the community services that were available. Up to the age of fifty, I was employed as a problem-shooter in engineering tasks. I believe that all problems are human. So, when I had problems I always looked for the answers from within myself. And mostly I found them. Once I recognised the kind of help Joyce required I would take the necessary action.

These days, I recognise more the need for help for myself. I have helped the local community services to train two specific home-help people. As a problem-shooter, I took the steps I needed to get some respite for myself.

Joyce spent a lot of time in the bedroom, especially when we were all home together. She began to talk to herself in the mirror. She always spent a bit of time making-up. Her eyebrows were rather bushy and she spent time plucking and shaping them. Gradually she developed a lack of co-ordination between hand and eyes. Her eyebrows began to look odd. Too thin in places and not very well shaped. She seemed to get irritated by the image in the mirror. One day she shaved her eyebrows off, and started using a lining pencil. This worked okay for quite a while. If she didn't like what she saw, she just washed it off and started again. Lipstick and pancake-type make-up became very liberally applied, especially under the chin and neck. Collars of blouses became smothered.

One day while we sat in the lounge, Joyce screamed from the bedroom 'This is MY HOUSE!! We thought she was rejecting our daughter. When it also happened in the bathroom and laundry, I realised that the mirrors were the problem. Re-orientation lasted about two minutes. She would kick and bang the mirror with her hands, repeating the 'This is MY HOUSE' scream. I painted all the mirrors white, peace in the house was regained.

Joyce went looking for 'that bloody woman' and found her down the street in the reflections in shop windows and cars. If a car stopped to let us cross the street, she would walk up to it and crash her hand on the windows, much to the consternation and dismay of the drivers.

The strange thing was that, now she could no longer see her face at home, she no longer wanted to or ever tried to use make-up again. I would line her eyebrows before taking her out, but gradually as her eyebrows grew again, I just simply stopped this practice. Her make-up is still on the dressing table, but she has no idea what it is for.

Joyce began to forget the logical order of many activities. It began one night when we went to bed and found there was a blanket in between the sheets.

We laughed.

'Oh dear!' she said. 'I've been silly.'

She had noticed the bed hadn't been made and had done it without my help.

This problem with logical order began to surface fairly rapidly over a period of a few weeks. I think it is a very clear example of the way that an activity that has started to deteriorate continues to do so with Alzheimer's disease. Handy hints to aid the sufferer are simply a stop-gap. Their use is restricted to a specific time during the deterioration of any activity.

Take the bed-making problem that I have just discussed. Let's devise a handy hint. We will have two sets of bedding prepared in the right order in large cardboard boxes. Put one away and let the sufferer make the bed using layers already put in the box in the right order so that when they are taken out the bed is made properly (that is, bottom sheet on the top etc.). When that set of bedding needs to be washed, the other box is brought into play. A reasonable solution?

Gradual deterioration soon makes the handy hint obsolete. The correct positioning of the bedding now becomes a problem. Too much hanging down one side: 'There's no sheet to tuck in!' on the other.

Handy hints, practical solutions must be tried at the right time; to do so too soon makes the sufferer even more aware of their disability and can cause trauma.

Dressing was also affected. Pants were put on over panty-hose. Pants were also put on back to front. Due to a slight but constant urine loss, Joyce always wore an adhesive sanitary pad. When she put her pants on back to front this affected the position of the pad. It became more frontal and very uncomfortable. She would wear a blouse and put her bra over the top. She became unable to select the right clothes to wear. She may wear her best dress for gardening, and wear one white shoe and a slipper. Dresses were worn back to front, and inside out, and she was no longer concerned about this.

The order of washing up and any cleaning became affected by the inability to remember the normal sequence. She was unable to mop the floor unless she cleaned ahead of herself, which meant she walked over the wet floor as she cleaned. The reason for this was simply that she could see what was ahead of her, but not what was behind. Her mind's eye could no longer perceive and recall what was behind. For Joyce, 'behind' no longer existed. Her range of vision became the limit of her ability. This then began to affect her ability to shower.

She would go into the shower and wash her hair first. She could put the shampoo into her hands and lift them to her head to apply shampoo, but, not being able to see the soap in her hair, she didn't rinse it out.

She kept the spray of water in front of her running from her breasts and down. She didn't wash her back or up between her legs. and she didn't dry the parts she couldn't see.

It seemed as if she were unable to feel that she was wet. She used to come out of the shower and put on her cotton dressing gown. Then it would be very noticeable that she hadn't dried herself because the back of the gown was wet and her hair was still soapy.

'Come here darling, let's go back into the shower and I'll help you,' I would say with a kiss.

Love, love and more love

So, that was that, I began to wash and shower her. This was at the beginning of 1988.

This was quite okay until Joyce's sexuality began to be affected. Prior to this, I was able to soap her all over, especially between the buttocks and in the vaginal area, and she was quite happy for me to do this. After a few months, she began to resist getting washed properly. At the same time, she lost her normal sexuality, her desire and of course, her sensuousness. This led to the cessation of our normal sexual relationship, but not of our sleeping together.

The problem with washing was solved by using the bath. I fill it to just over three-quarters full and put in plenty of bubbles. She is quite content to allow me to undress her, happily gets into the bath and has a good soak.

Occasionally, I put a wooden stool in the water and rest her feet on this to cut her toe-nails while she is in the bath. So I became a podiatrist, and am still able to keep her 'squeaky clean'.

By the end of 1988, Joyce could no longer read, write or communicate. Her speech in the main is unintelligible, although several times a day she comes to me and says, 'I do love you.'

She still does have an occasional realisation that something is wrong, and she liberates this by shouting, screaming and threats.

'I'll kill you,' she says.

'What for?' I ask.

'I don't know,' is the sad reply.

I also had to cope with Joyce's incontinence. She had had a long standing problem with a urine drip which had been only partially rectified by surgery. She also came to suffer from incontinence of the bowels. At first, I noticed that she did not flush toilet. Having emptied her bowels, she would simply forget that she had been on the toilet. Then, I noticed the absence of toilet paper in the unflushed toilet. Joyce would still wipe herself, but, having forgotten where to put well-used toilet paper, she would hide it.

Next she began to forget to wipe herself. Bed sheets and pants were regularly soiled. Finally, there came the stage where she simply forgot where to go. A bucket and shovel seemed the only realistic solution. I did try to help her find where to go with signs. Joyce sometimes gets to the toilet, but goes on floor. I am told this is a problem of perception.

For me, love, love and more love was the special ingredient required to overcome this.

Now, in 1990, what of Joyce ten years down the track? She spends most of her time pacing up and down. We bought her a doll for Christmas. She talks to it and loves it. She eats well, but uses only a spoon. I cut up her meat. If you give her a fork as well as a spoon, she becomes confused. She likes to carry something in her hand, be it a clothes peg, an article of clothing, a knife, or whatever. On 7 April, she turned sixty-three.

I take her to church on Wednesday mornings. She became disruptive on Sundays. The small congregation during the week are very understanding.

Knowledge is acceptance

What of me?   In the first few years when lack of knowledge prevented a true understanding, I went through all the stages of grief many times. It's a bit like being on a ladder. At the top is the peak of one's personal ambitions. Some make it, others reach a height that is satisfactory to them when they accept that that is about as far as they can get.

When Alzheimer's disease strikes, it becomes a downward climb which cannot be reversed. In the beginning, a step downwards is followed by a step up. The abilities of the sufferer seem all right most of the time.

Later, it's three steps down for every one up. These are the sufferer's peaks of concentration and attention, and can, unfortunately, give the carer the impression that things are really better.

It was during these steps that I went through different stages of grief. I was angry. I didn't believe what was happening. Sometimes, I was anxious or taken by self-pity. There was acceptance of a particular stage reached and re-adjustment.

'We're quite OK now. Perhaps, it will stay like this. I can manage this OK!'

Of course, it doesn't stay like this. Four steps down and two up.

Perhaps that's why my story focuses on the early stages of Alzheimer's disease. I noticed that once any activity started to deteriorate, it continued to do so until Joyce could no longer do it. I suspect that, although all sufferers are different, the same rule applies.

In my opinion, the best thing that any medical practitioner can do, if he or she suspects possible dementia, is to advise the carer immediately. Do not wait to be sure, for by that time the patient will be on the autopsy table. Tell the carer there is a possibility that the patient could have an irreversible disease of the brain. Further tests and observations may disprove that. I wish I had known earlier about how the deterioration of memory might affect the patient.

Taking into consideration the carer's condition or attitude as a reason for not telling them is not really helpful. If it is true that the patient has progressive dementia, the carer is going to find out in any case, the hard way. If the possible diagnosis is later disproved, then the carer will be happy. If not, then the carer will be prepared.

For me, understanding had to come first. Then, there was acceptance and finally the ability to cope. I feel it would be the same for most people.

In conclusion, I must tell you that Joyce and I, as members of the Anglican Church, visited the geriatric ward of the local hospital for a number years. We held hands with those unfortunates limited to staring into space, walked with the pacers, and talked with the uncertain. How amazing that we did not know what was wrong. Now we do.

Ern: Faith and love

The first indications that something was wrong with Dorothy was
a series of domestic disturbances, along with a severe decline in
general health, weight loss and rather unnatural behaviour —
suspicion, mainly about me, that I had interest in someone else, and
of others in the family, that things were being cooked up against
her. She even expressed concern about all those girls that I taught
at Senior Technical College, especially if I came home later than
usual.

Dorothy had been driving her own car for about thirteen years.
One day when we were out shopping she said, 'What gear am I in?'
This was in heavy traffic on the highway and I knew by the sound
of the motor that it wasn't top gear, so I told her to put her clutch
in and I changed gears for her. When we stopped at the lights she
said, 'Where's first?' My concern increased.

That would have been when Dorothy was about sixty-two, but
there were many similar occasions over a period of some years.

The earlier days

Prior to Dorothy's diagnosis in January 1984, we were holidaying
in our van on our daughter's property on the Sunshine Coast. A
mini-cyclone swept the area for two days and nights. I knew
Dorothy wasn't well and have often wondered how she managed
that ordeal so well. There was water literally crashing down on our
van, and thunder and lightning in frightening rapidity. Our annexe
nearly blew away, threatening to overturn the van. We didn't sleep
that night and, in a small lull in the storm when daylight came, we
managed to get the annexe off the van and then went into the house

for some relief. That night we slept inside the house and I recall my wife climbing into my bed like a frightened child as the storm continued. She was sure we were in a hospital and was very agitated. It took some extra doses of medication to get home to the south from that trip in 1983.

We were living in a two-storey house at that time and Dorothy had several falls, falling up the stairs, down the stairs. She fell out of the RV at home. For no apparent reason, she would black out. All of this was rather mysterious until I saw her have a bad turn while still in bed one morning. I called the doctor to whom I could only explain it as an epileptic seizure. He began treating her on this basis and the problem did not recur, although she did have some falls while in the geriatric hospital on respite. The doctors then said they were due to a series of minor strokes from which she recovered quite quickly with no physical damage except a black eye where she had fallen against a doorway.

On a lighter note, I noticed that her name was written on her dentures while she was in the hospital and remarked on this to the hospital staff.

The nurse said, 'Oh yes, we had to do that because someone put all the patients' teeth in a bowl for cleaning and they weren't named.'

When Dorothy first stayed at that hospital, she saw another lady sitting down crying and said, 'Oh, the poor thing!'

She went to her saying, 'Never mind dear! The Lord knows *all* about it!' and took her for a walk down the ward, holding her arm. They came back in good spirits.

The doctor, when approached, did some quick physical checks, then asked her some questions, which she was unable to answer. He gave her a referral to a neurologist, who ordered a brain scan.

The neurologist said the results showed positive brain deterioration.

'Dead cells, and there is nothing we can do with medicines or treatment. It happens to some of us earlier than others.'

No name was put to the diagnosis and the GP repeated the story when we went back to him. Not until two years later, when we saw a different doctor at our clinic, who asked, 'What about Alzheimer's?' was the diagnosis made clear. I realise now this was two years lost in adjustment time for me and in finding methods of coping.

Some incidents in our experiences would be typical of other Alzheimer sufferers. In the earlier days, while we still tried to enjoy our RV trips, we stayed at parks. When my wife went to the restroom, I would go and wait nearby for her, night or day. This was because she usually went in the opposite direction on leaving the block, especially if there were two entrances.

This was embarrassing at times, so I would speak to women passing on occasions and say, 'My wife has a memory problem. Would you mind checking on her?' I would describe her appearance, and there was virtually always co-operation.

On one of these occasions, in a park that was new to us, I waited and waited for her. I checked back at the van: no sign of her there. I approached the park manager and told him my story. He got a couple of people to assist me in a search, first of the toilets, and then around the park, with no success. I finally found her waiting at the van, oblivious of any problem. I hurriedly called off the search.

Another time she got into the wrong van, quite sure it was ours. Fortunately, the owners had noticed her confusion and brought her to the right van.

Wandering was also a problem. My wife would disappear from home at the first chance. When it first happened I combed the area in my car, with helpers out also, and a police car. She had put on extra clothes and a fur coat, and with her handbag, got a few blocks up the road. A lady saw her confusion and took her to the local police station. They phoned me. Apparently, she had some identification in her handbag — a necessity in these cases. There were more episodes of wandering, until I built a set of driveway gates secured with a combination lock which frustrated her attempts to 'go and see Mom'. Mom had died some twenty years ago. At least, the gates allowed me to relax a little.

Dorothy's obsession to 'go and see Mom' was very prominent in our experiences. It probably stemmed from the fact that her father died during the depression at the age of forty, when she was only six, at the younger end of a family of seven. So her mom did the massive job of raising the whole family alone. Even the older boys had trouble getting work: everything centred on Mom, a battler of diminutive size. She made a tremendous impression on my wife and also on the rest of the family.

Coping with this new person

For the first three years I coped without a break, or any outside help, doing everything — cooking, cleaning, washing, ironing, as well as supervising my wife's showering, toileting, choice of clothes and dressing, the latter after I discovered at times that she was wearing multiples of each garment.

Coping with this new person who couldn't reason or recall and retain anything new proved very difficult.

As a carer, I would like to express my appreciation of the nurses who came to our home at this stage and assisted with my wife's needs. Showering, shampooing her hair, and keeping a professional eye on her physical condition, as well as having a quick coffee and a chat, not only relieved the pressure on me, but made my day on many occasions, and reassured me when health problems occurred.

Also of great help were the breaks I had when Dorothy went to day care sessions, at first from ten until three in the afternoon, twice a week, and later two days weekly from four until eight in the evening, which included tea. I must admit I felt reluctant about letting her go to day care at first. But when time passed and her condition deteriorated, I found it to be an answer to the long days when I got pretty desperate. Most days she enjoyed the company. There were the sing-songs and games, and simple occupations like knitting squares which seemed to help her recall some old skills. There were a few times when she became very frustrated and agitated, and appeared relieved when I came to take her home.

Often with the help of medication, this was forgotten by the time we reached the house.

I tried to maintain my own expressions and demonstrations of love and affection, which seldom failed to calm her agitation and distress. It seemed to be the only positive factor in the confused state of her mind. 'I'm all upside down and inside out' was a frequent statement.

Many times, I have had to exercise my faith in God's ability to help us both, and calm the storm as He did long ago when He spoke 'Peace, be still' to the waves. I would see my wife go to sleep like a child.

However, the years of caring twenty-four hours in every day took their toll. I am thankful for the measure of health and strength I had, and for my ability to do the necessary chores for us both. It was important for me to maintain the meticulous standards which my wife had kept, but I developed stomach and digestive problems which the doctor said was 'everything to do with it' — my caring problems!

Respite and a fellow feeling

After about three years, respite breaks of a month, twice a year, helped. This increased to three times a year as the pressure built up.

Finally, an opportunity arose for my wife's long-term care in a special purpose hostel for Alzheimer's sufferers. I only agreed to this after considerable pressure from family, doctors and the staff at the geriatric hospital, who had provided referrals to suitable hostels.

Then, of course, there were other adjustments to be made, living apart after forty-nine years of marriage, knowing that your partner now shared residency with nine others in a similar condition to herself.

The staff at the hostel are caring and understanding and do their best to make the residents comfortable and at home. It's a mammoth task and we are grateful to them.

The inevitable thoughts arose in this situation.

'Could I have hung on a bit longer?'

'Did I do the right thing?'

'How long before another opportunity would arise?'

'Will she be given enough loving care?'

There were feelings of guilt and grieving at the loss of a loved one, though I had had them since the effects of the disease made it apparent that my smart, loving, meticulous girl was no more and could not remember being married to me nearly fifty years before, or even what my name was.

I find it difficult to understand what it must feel like to live without a memory, because the brain itself is in a tangled mess and much of it has ceased to function anyway. The last learned skills of a lifetime are the first to be lost and forgotten. Then, it progresses backwards to childhood abilities but without any of the ability to learn as a child does. You become increasingly dependent on your carer to understand you and provide for your needs, health and safety.

I found that trying to enter into these problems makes one very sensitive to every indication the sufferer can give to tell you of their needs, fears and concerns because communication breaks down as the disease progresses.

Hallucinations add to Dorothy's agitation and distress. She often starts off to tell you a story about what they said and did, and is very sincere and obviously convinced they are real, but I never get to know what it is all about.

My wife's greatest pleasure and occupation is discussing at length with her friend in the mirror, when she pulls up a chair and spends hours talking about their common interests. But the conversation goes wrong when they apparently disagree or tell her off. She becomes very disturbed and agitated, and distraction is often the only way to break the sequence. I try 'Come and have a cup of tea!' or perhaps 'Would you like a walk around the block?'

A small dose of helpful medication sometimes succeeds in getting her back to some reality.

I found that in these situations I needed friends with whom I could chat in an outgoing manner to relieve the tensions that build up. I think, in fact, that they are hard to find as it seems evident that those who have been through the same or similar traumatic experiences have the best understanding of the needs of the carer him/herself.

Even a quick phone call can break the tension sequence for that day; a word of encouragement has great value. It's great to be able to talk sensibly with intelligent people who are on the outside of your situation and can bring themselves into it by their genuine interest.

On the other hand, it's not hard to pick those who enquire from politeness, but tend to switch off when you begin to tell them the true position. 'Fellow feeling does make us wondrous kind!'

Probably the worst problem I had to deal with personally as a carer was the intolerance that builds up. Not with my girl, as I call Dorothy — to her pleasure, and I still love her very much — but with the disease which has wrought such havoc.

One answer which proved effective for me was a quickly arranged respite break during which I managed a bus tour holiday and came home quite refreshed with a lot of fresh memories to think about.

I have known carers who are desperate for a break, for some relief in an unanswerable situation, but this has been denied them.

A relative in her late seventies and with poor health herself, battled on caring for her husband. He had had several small strokes and other health problems and didn't seem to notice what was being done for him or at what cost until she entered a hospital and died within two weeks.

I felt I had lost a good pal, someone I could phone or call on at any time to discuss our mutual problems and share any humour we saw in our situation. We were able to express our mutual faith in the One who could help us most. You can say an effectual prayer over the phone!

Another friend of long standing contacted me when she heard of my wife's sickness. She had recently lost her husband, also my friend from early days. Again, we have built up an understanding based on mutual support and in the expression of our feelings, and of the reactions and tensions felt in the grieving for our loved ones. It does help to know that someone else understands your feelings and has experienced what you are going through. Such good friends certainly had an answer to the loneliness that I sometimes experienced.

I have also enjoyed an involvement in art, having commenced oil painting in the year before retirement. It was important for me to have some satisfaction from a creative hobby. Combined with photography on holiday trips and the ability to produce my own picture frames, it occupied any spare time available during the caring years and provided a therapy as well.

When she was well enough to travel, my wife and I spent some time each year, as mentioned earlier, on extended vacations, until the disease caused deterioration and led to an inability to take long driving trips. And so we parted with another of our retirement pleasures. Even the photos do not recall those pleasures for her now.

So now Dorothy and I live apart because of this great separator, Alzheimer's disease. It's degenerative and we cannot expect more than occasional days out together. I can visit at any time, providing nothing disrupts the task of the caring staff.

It appears to be very important for a carer to be always buoyant in spirit, not to seem worried but to be always in control of any situation that may concern the sufferer. The carer needs a lot of answers!

It may be that my wife is very sensitive but she picks up my mood or attitude very quickly, often making me wish that I hadn't spoken or shown my feelings in her presence. It then takes some time to convince her that everything is all right and she has no need to worry.

Legal and money matters

Dorothy has not handled money for years and has lost all sense of its value. If I mention that I have a bill to pay for $100, for example, she usually says, quite concerned, 'Oh dear, I haven't got that much.'

My usual answer is, 'I have. I'll fix it.'

Whereupon, I get a kiss and, 'You're a good boy!' Even such a small gesture of thanks and some sign of appreciation do help, and certainly boost morale!

Getting a place in a special purpose hostel is one thing, it is another to finance it. For patients without assets, no ingoing payment is required. However, a sliding scale defines the contribution required.

A monthly rental of eighty-five per cent of the aged pension is often payable, plus fifty per cent of any other income the patient may have. The marital home is not included in the assets for this purpose when there is a spouse living and requiring accommodation. I am trying to sell our home to cover the cost of the contribution. This meant a considerable upheaval of my domestic and financial situation but will occupy some of the early separation period, and help tide me over the adjustments.

The legal and proper administration of a disabled person's affairs by another requires an enduring power of attorney. This includes a person who by reason of a brain disease, like Alzheimer's, is no longer capable of making decisions, or reasoning out or understanding financial business or property transactions. To be legal, this is better obtained from the person while they have the understanding and, therefore, the capacity to consent to and execute it. Failing this, a spouse, family member or interested close friend can apply for a hearing to appoint a suitable administrator to attend to the incapacitated person's needs in these matters and to act in the person's interests. The administrator is responsible to the board and must obtain the board's approval and consent to any property transactions and for certain investments on the disabled person's behalf. It is also necessary to present accounts of their dealings with the person's financial affairs.

Faith in a time of need

Through all of this my faith has been a great support for me. When I look back over all the events of the past several years, a passage from the Letter to the Hebrews wells up in my memory and reminds me that we have the assurance of a Great High Priest who is touched with the feelings of our infirmities, to whom we can appeal at any time, and from whom we 'find grace to help in time of need'. (Hebr.4)

Judith: 101 ways to make a bed

Caring for Mom over the last two years, I have found to be a very stressful and tiring time. I really feel for those who care for their loved ones for years on end. Looking back I can see that Mom was very clever in covering up her dementia for as long as she did. Knowing what I now know, there were quite a few tell-tale signs but being inexperienced with Alzheimer's disease, we were unable to recognise them.

Tell-tale signs

The first important thing that comes to mind is the day when we visited Mom to find her very upset because Telecom had sent a letter saying her phone would be disconnected if the account wasn't paid. She was sure that she had paid it but couldn't find the receipt. Mom had always been very particular about paying her accounts on time, so this was evidently the start of her forgetting things.

We lived one hundred miles away and at this time I was working full-time. Our eldest son was working out of state, our daughter and other son were also working, but living at home. My husband and I could manage a visit only once a week to see Mom. Even then I wasn't always able to get the days off, so my husband would go by himself to check with her.

I rang each day to ask what she was having for lunch and the answer was always a well-prepared menu. However, we soon realised she was not eating properly: her cooking and eating habits were all in her memory. We arranged to have meals on wheels delivered for her (against her wishes), but thankfully, when they arrived she accepted them for about six months. Then each time we called we gradually found more and more meals stowed away, untouched.

We also noticed that Mom was getting very careless with her housekeeping and particularly her personal hygiene, which was not like her at all. So it was necessary to bath and change her each time we called. I took all her washing home and returned it on the next visit. I would put the clean clothes, including sheets, towels, and the rest on her spare bed.

Each week she would say the same thing, 'I have done the washing, but haven't got around to putting it away as yet.'

Each time we called we faced something different. Maybe it was a hide-and-seek game looking for her handbag. Believe me, it turned up in such unexpected places, it's no wonder she couldn't find it herself.

She would take all the keys out of the doors, even the wardrobe keys, and they would be stowed away anywhere. She lost the back-door key, then attacked the lock with a hammer. She then called to say someone had broken into the house and there was no peace until we were able to get up there to do the necessary repairs. After that we attached the key by a chain to each appropriate door. The wardrobe-door keys were removed altogether.

Then there were the bricks piled up at the back door to be put against it at night. There were pieces of wood and long sticks beside the bed, a whistle (which didn't work) was under her pillow. Again, looking back, I realise she must have felt very insecure which was not like Mom at all.

'...a woman of her age'

Along the way, my sister and I had both spoken to Mom's doctor, and said we were concerned at her actions and thought she was getting very forgetful. He brushed us off and said there was nothing wrong, just the normal progress for a woman of her age. She was seventy-nine-years-old.

Eventually we took over the payment of all Mom's accounts as she would forget them or worse still, try to pay them twice. At the same time, she was going to her neighbour for so many things that this kindly woman was also getting very concerned about Mom's actions. She couldn't turn the gas heater on, so the same neighbour or one of her children would go in and do it for her. They would hardly be back in their own home and she would be there to ask them to turn the heater off. Then it was the same procedure with the light switches. Often the outside lights were left on all night. One day, she was out in the yard only partly dressed, so again it was that caring neighbour who came to the rescue and went in and got her dressed properly. Without this wonderful woman's help, we would have had more trouble earlier than we did.

Despite all these things, Mom still insisted she was quite capable of looking after herself. Any mention of even coming to us for a holiday met with very strong resistance.

Small incidents come to mind: trying to convince Mom that a vase of flowers was artificial — even when we pulled one flower apart and showed her the wires and other parts, she turned around, looked at us and said, 'Those flowers have lasted so well. You know, I grew those roses!' Her neighbour also told us that she had caught Mom lighting matches under the electric kettle.

After twelve months, we realised that things were much worse at each visit and we felt it wasn't safe to leave Mom on her own any longer. We were faced with a very difficult decision. I was lucky to have my husband, so understanding and supportive at all times.

My sister, who lives out of state, couldn't believe how bad Mom had become since she last saw her. She usually visited twice a year, staying each time, about ten days. To her, Mom was still okay, just a bit forgetful, so that when I said that my husband and I felt she should not be left on her own and that we had decided to take her to live with us, my sister insisted that if anything happened to Mom through the move, we would have to accept full blame for it. She reasoned that Mom had lived in her own home for forty-odd years and that to move her now would cause her to fret and die.

I knew that if she stayed on her own, she would starve to death, die from neglect or might even set fire to the house while she was inside. I pointed out a few more things: pegs in the refrigerator, tea-leaves in the kettle, outside rubbish bin in the kitchen, or buckets of sheep manure on the porch. There were so many little things: but my sister still wasn't convinced.

What to do next?

Our decision made, we packed a bag for Mom and told her she needed a holiday. Surprisingly, this time she was quite happy to come with us. She thought it was only for a little while.

Even with all this concern, we managed to make the necessary arrangements for my daughter's wedding. Mom being only about four feet eight inches in height and a kind and gentle natured person, all the wedding guests thought she was wonderful. My eldest son danced with her throughout the night and we have the wedding on video, so we will always have a happy memory of Mom doing and enjoying something she loved.

My daughter and her husband went off on their honeymoon, so we had her moving out of home one week, and Mom moving in the next. This was the immediate problem solved, but now we had her with us, what were we to do next?

After days of talking about the best way to approach the situation, nights of little sleep, and weeks of trying to convince family and friends whom we thought could help us, to do so, we realised we were on our own and left with the responsibility to do what we felt was best for Mom.

We found we were unable to leave Mom alone in the house as she was having trouble finding her own bedroom. My doctor suggested I have a geriatric assessment done. We were told she probably had Alzheimer's disease. For a while, we weren't too sure what to do or who to turn to for help. Eventually, I decided to leave work and look after Mom. What a decision! I sometimes felt I had taken on more than I was capable of, but somehow with help from my husband I managed.

My doctor again suggested I contact the local council. 'They should have any information you need for help.' I'm afraid I was disappointed. However, my ex-boss rang me one day to see how we were getting on and asked me if I had tried help from a day care center. She gave me a contact number to ring and this was one of the best things I ever did. The sister in charge of the center arranged for Mom to go there for a few hours one day, to see if she liked it and was able to cope. It worked out fine. She went for one day a week and after a time, it was two days and eventually three days each week. Those days at the center proved to be my lifesavers — some days I was so tired that I felt ready to give in, but after each break I was able to keep going.

The emotional ties

The twelve months during which I looked after Mom in my own home were, at times, very depressing. My feelings were confused: I thought I was either coping very well, or not doing as well as I should be.   I'm sure it would be easier to manage the practical, day-to-day tests of patience if there was any way to get rid of the emotional ties.

My life now was mainly spent looking after Mom. I attended carers meetings every second week which made me realise I was not on my own. We shared a few tears on occasions, but we also laughed together. I also realised that even though at times I felt I had had a terrible day, someone else would relate the tale of a day which seemed worse than mine. The group also provided good practical advice about how to lift people from baths and the like. This was a source of real help and support.

Seeing Mom deteriorate each day, losing yet another skill that she'd had for so many years, was very difficult to accept. My daughter one day said to me, 'You know, Mom, Nanna is no longer living, she is only existing.' My older boy had difficulty in coming to terms with what was happening. He confided, 'Nanna taught me to play cards, along with so many other things, and now she can't even play the simplest of card games.' My younger son best seemed to accept what was happening, perhaps because he was home all the time, which made it easier for him to adjust gradually as time went by.

The progress of Mom's condition made it easier for my sister and me to sort ourselves out, and she agreed that she had now accepted the situation as it was.

The doctor who saw Mom for the geriatric treatment advised me to talk to Mom about enduring power of attorney, while she was still able to consent to this. This wasn't easy to do: my mother had been telling *me* what to do for so many years. I had to reverse the roles and realise that I was now responsible for her well-being, almost as if I were her parent. But I am grateful that I took the doctor's advice and had this done then because it wasn't long after that there was quite a change.

Mom's span of concentration was lessening each day and she was very confused at times. We went through the trauma of selling her property, and with it came the realisation that she'd never be able to use most of her belongings and personal effects again. I could not bring myself to dispose of them while she was alive so we bundled them up and stored them.

Again, my wonderful husband did so much of the cleaning up and running around. It just seemed unfair for him to have to do so much but there were only the two of us. One good thing did come out of all this: it made us have a good clean-up at home and get rid of a lot of unnecessary rubbish. We vowed never to hoard again.

Loss of skills

When Mom first came to live with us, she was still able to do a few odd jobs without any help, but almost daily we could see her failing. After a time, her idea of washing dishes was to run them under the tap, often using only cold water. Then she would dry them off, dirt and all. This resulted in my making sure I did all the washing up while she dried. I persevered with this arrangement, but at times it got very frustrating. She would decide she had finished and hang the tea towel up in the middle of it all. She would dry the dishes and put them back into the dish rack. Sometimes she put them on the bench and moved each article around, drying each one three or four times. Some nights it was a very long task!

Sweeping the floor became another worry. Mom ended up pushing the dirt around the floor, unable to pick it up or even get it into a pile. She also lost the skill of folding clothes and would roll them instead. In the end, she could not even pair the socks. I made up a basket of clothes that were no longer being worn and she was happy to fold these, sometimes two or three times a day. This way, I didn't have the worry of her making more work for me.

Some days were more difficult than others. Mom would constantly want to help and I would have trouble finding something she was able to do. All this time, she was still convinced that she was able to care for herself. This could be very hard to take, especially when I had just been through the process of showering and dressing her.

Around this time, I'm sure I could have written a book titled 'One Hundred and One Ways to Make a Bed'. You can't imagine the way her bed turned out some days!

As time went by, I found I had to be very explicit in what I told her as she was having difficulty with all tasks. The daily process was much the same, and I found while I could keep to a routine it was okay. But the least upset and she didn't know where she was.

I was able to get two weeks respite care, which was a relief for all concerned. Even my patient husband enjoyed the short break. Our younger son remarked how quiet it was without Nanna. When I said that Nanna didn't make any noise, he said, 'No, that's true, but you certainly do a lot of yelling when she is here.' I made up my mind that I should not lose my cool when Mom came home. My intentions were good but I just couldn't put them into practice.

It may be coincidence but after Mom came home from respite care she seemed to be on a downhill run again. I remarked on this to the sister in charge of the day care center. She said that they had noticed that Mom was getting more confused but that it was just a general decline.

From then on, everything I said had to be repeated over and over before Mom could grasp what had to be done. Just getting her dressed or undressed was tiring. One day I said to her, 'Mom, put this dress on and we will go and do some shopping.' She got the dress on, but over the clothes she was already wearing at the time.

Another day, I had her dressed in all but her cardigan. I left her for only a few minutes and when I got back she had her legs in the sleeves. To get her dressed now it was a case of 'Put your leg in here, put your foot in your slipper, put your arm in here.' And quite often I had to simply put her feet or arms just where they were needed. To get her to go to the toilet, or for me to clean her teeth, tried the little patience I had left.

We found that Mom was having little naps off and on all day while sitting in her chair, so that when she went to bed, she was only sleeping a couple of hours each night. Often she was out of bed getting clothes on again and we hadn't even got into bed. It was nothing now for her to be out of bed eight or nine times a night, always bumping into things or knocking articles off her chest of drawers. Eventually all that she had in her room was her bed and the chest. I had to remove all other items for her own safety.

My younger son and my husband were also disturbed each time I was out of bed to see what Mom was up to. They were going off to work looking tired before the day had started for them, and I was irritable most mornings as well. But not Mom; she came out with her usual remarks, 'I had a lovely cosy sleep last night, didn't hear a sound all night!' If only I had been able to tell her differently!

The next plan

I delayed the next plan of action as long as I could. Eventually, I consulted the doctor to see if he could give Mom something to help her sleep better. We tried two different tablets — but it was just like feeding her candy: she was still out of bed at three or four in the morning.

On the next visit to the doctor for a consultation about tablets, it was decided that it was also time for the doctor to fill in the nursing home admission form to keep it current. When he had done so, he turned to me and said, 'Your mother is ready for full-time nursing care.'

I felt the same confusion as when I had found out that she had Alzheimer's disease. I just didn't know which way to turn, or who to go to for help. I spoke to the day care sister again and she sent me to the welfare officer connected to the nursing home associated with the day care center. She was very kind and after speaking with her, I now felt at least I knew what I had to do to get Mom into a nursing home.

Knowing what to do was one thing, getting a position for Mom was another. From the list of nursing homes that the welfare officer gave me, I found that ninety per cent didn't even have a waiting list. There were just too many people needing care. I had previously made a general enquiry at a nursing home that had recently been built near where my sister lived. No waiting list applied, so I decided to see if they had any vacancies. I was told they gave preference to people living in the area, but they were very understanding and said that, seeing Mom's other daughter lived in the area, they would keep her in mind if a vacancy did show up.

In only a week I received a phone call. I asked if I could have time to gather my thoughts and after talking with my husband and this time, my sister also, we decided that we had to accept the position at least and see how Mom coped with the new environment.

After a panic to get her bits and pieces together and as many of her clothes named as we could, we arrived three days later at the nursing home. It was really more like hostel style accommodation. Mom had her own room with bathroom en suite and her own furniture and furnishings. She appeared to settle in quite well.

Four weeks down the track, I began to feel so good in myself. I made up my mind to go back to work part-time and get my life back together again. I felt that the last two years were a phase that cannot be forgotten but also not a time for me to dwell on. I felt again so much love for Mom. I didn't have that constant concern I felt near the end of the time she was with us, that my love was turning to resentment.

I also felt quite sure that we had done as much as we were able to do, and now was the time to get the necessary help to make Mom's days easier for her. We were just not able to keep going twenty-four hours a day.

I didn't feel guilty about the decision to place Mom in a nursing home, rather perhaps there was the guilt of feeling so relieved that the burden had been taken from us.

Aftermath

It is now four months since we made the decision to place Mom in a nursing home and what a decision it has proved to be. I thought my stress and anxiety would ease but instead, at times, the increase is unbelievable.

We knew the nursing home was opposed to a locked environment, but didn't realise this would prove to be such a hassle. Mom had been accepted with the knowledge of her Alzheimer's disease, and of her wandering, but they didn't seem to be able to accommodate this. The person in charge didn't appear to understand Alzheimer's disease. They try to treat these patients as you would the frail aged and don't accept that their needs are different.

During one of our visits to Mom, while we sat out on the verandah enjoying the sunshine, in less than one hour the staff came running out three times to rescue one of the other women who was making her way to the front gate. A safety lock on the gate would enable patients to have the freedom of the front yard and stop anxious moments and wasted time.

I still feel we made the right decision in placing Mom in a nursing home, although perhaps the choice wasn't a good one. We took advantage of the position available because we intended to move there next year and we wanted to avoid yet another move for Mom. The distance has been a concern because the number of trips we have had to make.

Many phone calls from the management were to tell me that Mom was wandering, that she doesn't sleep well at night, and once, that my mother needed twenty-four-hour care!! If we had been able to give that constant care Mom would still be at home with us. Management agreed that they accepted Mom knowing these things, but they also felt she should have settled in more quickly. Several times I felt they were telling us to find another place.

I rang the Alzheimer's Disease and Related Disorders Society. They were understanding and helpful and gave me a contact number for information on nursing homes where I was given the names of three other homes in the same area and told that they could also help with urgent placement if necessary. We really don't want to move her but if we have to, at least we have someone to go to for help.

After numerous trips to discuss Mom's behaviour, it was suggested on one occasion we pay extra for a companion as management felt that Mom was taking up too much of the staff's time. We agreed to pay an extra $100 per week, but after thinking more about this arrangement, we felt uneasy, that the cost could only increase as time went by and that we hadn't made the right decision. We rang the Health Department, to enquire about our position. They explained a few things and advised if we wanted to pay extra that was up to us, but they wouldn't recommend it.

The next day, I rang the Nursing Home and told them of our decision not to pay for a companion, and also that we had spoken with the Health Department. Our contact with the Department had promised a meeting with the administration staff of the nursing home. For a few weeks, I felt very concerned, as if we were at fault and were stirring up trouble. However, when speaking to each party separately, they both reassured me everything was okay and that they would sort things out with no ill feelings.

In spite of the management's promise to keep in touch with us, at this stage the only calls were when I rang to enquire how Mom was. Each time I received a favourable report on her progress. On one occasion, I felt I was getting a school report on one of my children, the details of improvement and the way Mom had settled in were difficult to accept.

After a few more phone calls and yet another visit to discuss Mom's behaviour, the matter now seems to be under control.

During our last visit to the nursing home, even though the atmosphere was tense, I felt the outcome of the meeting was positive. The report was that Mom had settled down and her wandering, for the moment anyway, had improved.

They have tried several medications and have found one to help Mom sleep through the night. She looks very well and shows no sign of anxiety when we leave, and I am now quite happy with the care she is receiving.

I am also feeling better in myself again after that last visit, and hope to be able to settle down now and relax knowing all is well with Mom at last. It will soon be Christmas and before I know it we will be busy getting ready to move.

Writing about some of my experiences in caring for a mother with Alzheimer's disease has helped me greatly by relieving a lot of built-up tension. I hope that someone reading this will gain from what I have written and perhaps write some of their own experiences to find relief in the same way.

There is no way I could have coped with this troubled period in my life without the help and support of my family, especially my wonderful husband, who has driven me thousands of miles to visit Mom. He has been my strength and comfort. I also value the support from the people at the day care center, and the carers group, which I still attend each fortnight.

I can't change anything that has passed and so now I look forward to what I hope will be a happy and less stressful time in my life, which I intend to enjoy.

John & Meg: Twenty beers before dinner

The scenario

Jimmy South went looking for John. It was out of character for John to miss two shifts.

John was a two-shift man, a hardworking foreman on the wharf. He liked his work and often did overtime. His home life was quiet; he and his wife had parted years before. Working and drinking, working and drinking, these two things filled John's days.

Jimmy found John at home, asleep under his elevated house. John had no idea how long he'd been there. He had locked himself out of the house and was unable to find the keys. He didn't know where his car was. He was unkempt, unshaven and had no food in the house, only alcohol. Jimmy took John to the hospital.

John's admission notes record that he was unsteady on his feet, lethargic, disinterested in eating, and very vague. He did not know the day, date, year, or even where he lived. The diagnoses given were Wernicke's encephalopathy and Korsakoff's psychosis.

The next two months are a mystery to John, even now, two years down the track. John's only recollections are 'panic and utter loneliness'.

The alcohol and poor eating habits of years had taken their toll. For a time it appeared that John would need to give up almost all of his independence and live in supervised accommodation. He needed assistance to find his bed in the ward, and had no insight into his memory problems. He also had what the occupational therapist noted as lack of intent. Midway through a task he would forget what he was doing.

With good nutrition, copious amounts of sleep, and occupational therapy, John recovered many of his old skills. After six weeks he was able and motivated to dress, groom, wash and feed himself. Two areas of functioning remained problems; John's short-term memory was very poor and he could not learn new information. This meant he frequently got lost in the ward and did not know what day, month or even what year it was. A hostel placement seemed to be indicated. But John was adamant. First, he wanted to go home. Second, he wanted to go back to work on the wharf. The first was marginally possible, the second not possible due to his memory problems.

With assistance from health and welfare service providers, it has proved possible for John to return home, and to live quite independently. For four days a week John works at a sheltered workshop where he sharpens wooden garden stakes. His manual skills and his verbal skills have earned him a place on the management committee. The other day of the working week is a day off. John attends a social group that caters especially for people with memory loss, he has a chance to socialise and he also meets Barbara, a Red Cross worker. She makes up a shopping list for John and together they do his weekly shopping. Red Cross also send a home care worker to John's house once a week to clean the floors and bathroom for him. A Red Cross gardener does the heavy gardening work.

John received superannuation and this is managed by the Public Trustee, who make a fortnightly transfer into his bank account.

He knows what to do each day and what day it is by using a diary. It's become his most important possession.

Meg's story
John is my Dad.

I became aware of his problem through a phone call from my step-mother in late 1988. She told me Dad had had some kind of episode due to his drinking. However, when I rang the hospital the nurse on duty told me it was a health problem and the alcohol that had brought about the collapse. The episodes are often caused by long bouts of malnourishment coupled with heavy drinking. So he really had two problems, nourishment and addiction.

My father had always been a drinker. From my earliest recollection I can distinctly see him with glass in hand. What I find unusual now is that he doesn't drink and can't remember drinking. As an indication of how much he could down in a day, I can remember instances where he would finish twenty cans before dinner and still have room for a nightcap, although he would be a little wobbly.

The alcohol affected his relationship with others; he was not a very tolerant man when I was younger. He could not deal with any infraction of his rules in any other way except to get angry. Towards the end of my parents' marriage, he became increasingly violent. We left in 1970. Dad remarried in the late seventies; I now have a half-sister and a new step-family.

We didn't keep in close touch. I didn't contact Dad until Christmas 1983. I used to move around so much that he would not have had any idea where I was living anyway.

When I finally got to see him in 1984, he was very flat. That's the only way I could describe it. Beforehand, he used to react to everything; by 1984, he was like a rag doll. He would come home from work, flop in front of the television, and that would be that. He seemed totally physically exhausted. He wasn't drinking inside the house, but he had booze stashed all over town, as I found to my amazement when visiting childhood friends. There was a carton on practically every corner.

Since the incident where he was found under the house, and my move back to the same city, things have changed again. He doesn't get so bad tempered, although changes to his plans upset him somewhat. He is definitely *not* the same person he was before the memory loss began.

Our relationship has changed as well. When we were living together as a family, Dad was extremely autocratic. One had to do as one was told, when one was told. The memory loss has made Dad very dependent, and I find myself more in the role of parent to him. In some senses, the roles have reversed completely: he is more like a child and I am the one who has to be autocratic. He has to be bullied into some tasks because he will insist that he has done them, even when it is patently obvious that he hasn't.

I realise now that Dad's memory was deteriorating even before 1988 (although it's stabilised now). I put it down to the booze. He would forget that I'd rung the week before or would not remember he was supposed to ring on such and such a day. He always seemed vague about what he was doing and tended to say the same thing as a way of passing the time. Often we would have these strange circular conversations without ever coming to any answers to my questions. I thought he might also have been going deaf.

After he was able to return to his home with the help of the wonderful Red Cross and Fiona, a very enthusiastic worker in the field of dementia, things got better. At first he did not want to record anything, even my phone calls, but Fiona insisted and he now is chained to his personal diary. He won't do anything without consulting it first.

I was living in Sydney at the time and found it difficult to keep up with what was going on but I noticed the improvement over the months. Dad's memory may not be what it was, but his ability to cope is returning. He doesn't seem as helpless as he once was. He also initiates things a little more than he did. The diary system has given him a portable reference system. It's as if his memory is now outside his brain and in his pocket. He is lost without it.

My father's confidence is gradually being restored although he does have some unrealistic expectations about transport. He cannot drive any more. I personally think he would be dangerous on the road, as his concentration sometimes lapses when he is performing tasks.

For instance, one night he decided to fix a radio for my stepmother. The radio was on top of the fridge, so instead of taking the radio off the fridge, he got a chair and stood on it. He *very* narrowly missed having the top of his head chopped off by the ceiling fan (which was on at the time).

He does tend to get depressed at times but can usually be snapped out of it by action of some sort. This leads me to believe that the depression's origins stem from lack of activity. In other words, he's bored.

He is reluctant to try new things, but actually enjoys them once he can be coaxed into doing then. Dad seems to need the security of having someone to oversee his actions. He is quite aware that his memory makes some tasks very difficult.

My father does not go out to see his friends very often, and tells me he feels sad when he sees them. I think his job was the only prop to his self-esteem that he had in his life before. Now he is having to construct other props.

As far as my daily routine goes, I've learned to disregard the order and the disorder. My father has a very strict routine from which he can't be disturbed especially in the morning. I found this very frustrating, as it was hard to be spontaneous, but I've come to accept that he needs that order.

For example, if I want to have breakfast on the verandah, Dad will become agitated because 'this isn't what you do in the morning. Afternoons are the proper time for the verandah'.

There was an incident in the city. Dad became very upset, disoriented and uncomfortable because it 'wasn't the sort of place one can relax in'.

If I want to go out by myself, I have to tell him 8000 times that I won't be home for tea. I usually leave several notes around to say where I will be, and I've put a white board on the fridge with all the days of the week clearly marked, again so he'll know where I am. The spontaneity has had to go, and a fair deal of planning goes into every day.

I also find myself double checking things like the iron and the stove (just to be sure). He sometimes gets up at night and wanders around aimlessly, but that is only when he's not exercised during the day. I wait for him to go back to bed because he can be very unsteady on his feet when he wakes up.

As far as choosing any one thing that helped confront Korsakoff's, I feel that the Red Cross people who came to help Dad after his hospital stay were the most helpful. They helped him orientate himself in time and space. Basically, they kept him in touch with the real world.

I was lucky to have my nursing background, because it was from there that I gained my understanding of what was happening to Dad, and of how to manage. I swapped notes with relatives of people at the nursing home where I was working, and found out how they handled similar problems.

Fiona has been a great support. She took me out for a few respite nights when I first re-visited town and saw my much changed father. It was a great comfort to know she had things in charge when I was so far away.

John's own story

To start, my daughter had to remind me that I had this task to do.

I did not realise I was forgetting things. My daughter speaks of me forgetting when she phoned as far back as 1986, but I did not recognise a memory problem.

Right up to the time I was found under the house, I was working. There were no complaints from either the wharfies or the management, as far as I can remember. After the episode of being found under the house and being hospitalised, I realised that my short-term memory was inadequate for commercial life.

This did, however, take a bit of pressure. It had to be pointed out to me that I was not remembering things as of yore, and it took quite a good deal of persuasion from people close to me to make me believe this.

There were a couple of incidents which shook me around a bit. Once I was at a park I know well, waiting to catch a bus, and I could not remember which side of the street I had to catch it from, let alone what number bus to catch. Now, I have the number written in my diary, and the bus drivers give me a whistle if I'm on the wrong side.

Another day, I looked down and found I had odd shoes on. I remember saying to myself, 'I've got another pair like that at home!'

I had to get into the habit of double checking everything. Had I shaved? Did I have clean clothes on? Had I fed the cats? Are all the appliances switched off? Do I have the door key in my pocket?

Even now, I sometimes tell myself it's a natural slowing down of a once too active brain. Resentment was my first reaction, resentment against most things in general. I live with that resentment. I haven't got over it. Occasionally I snap at people and I'm ashamed of that. Generally, I contain myself.

As for the hospital admission, it's like that part of my history is in cotton wool. Nothing is clear. My daughter reminds me that I thought I'd had a heart attack, or a brain lesion, or even a recurrence of war injuries. All I wanted was to go home.

Before the hospitalisation, I was the fellow in charge. I knew everything, all the answers. Now I don't know the questions. I have to smile, as other people tell me what to do. It's very hard to get used to. I think I'm managing it a bit better than, say, six months ago. That does not mean that I like it.

Talking to people hasn't seemed likely to be much help; no-one can understand. I've tried speaking to people at the Fire Escape which is a social group for people who have poor memories. That's all.

The workshop is more congenial than the wharf but there's no cut and thrust. I used to meet a lot of people, now you can't discuss much. Once you've discussed the point on a piece of timber, that's it. I don't really consider it to be work. The interaction on the wharf was beautiful. I could make those people move! There was one job to do and eight men, plus myself. That meant nine ways to do it! To get the job done was an art. Work was a lot more stimulating — interaction all the time.

To try to find a substitute for the stimulation I used to get at work, I've taken to reading much more. But, there again, it's just vicarious stimulation.

With Meg home now, we potter a bit. We've put up a trellis for some peas, and I work on the house a bit. I am ashamed to say I watch a lot more television.

Another change I've found difficult to adjust to is my lack of mobility. I used to have a car. Now I walk or take the bus, and I despise the bus. I am at the beck and call of others. I don't feel as free to move about. I have gone out walking and been lost, even though I used to know this area very well and I have practised certain routes many times.

Nowadays it's a big mental effort to go out at all. Getting lost and having to ask for directions was the sort of thing that led me to withdraw for a while. I didn't want to see anyone. I didn't seek out information. I coped by sitting down. I tended to minimise these difficulties to myself, but other people noticed. Eventually, the support of Fiona and, then, the people at the workshop got me going.

I had something to do there, and I saw people who were in much worse condition than myself. Being busy and seeing the others helped me get going.

The strategy that has helped me most is my diary. I'm getting closer to it every day. I get upset if the book is not to hand. There is an entry for every appointment and every day out. Each day, I put a tick beside the date, and I never go out without it. Words I have written are always there to go back to. It's a great help.

I go into a panic when I can't find my diary. Religiously, every morning, I get up and read what I did yesterday. Then, I list for today. If I feel my back pocket, and the diary is not there, it looks like I'm doing one of those West Indian dances. I swivel around, patting every pocket, and there's always a great sigh of relief when I find it.

Having a memory problem has changed my opinions about people. I never despised health workers and cleaning ladies, but I regarded them as minions before. Now I think they're really nice; they're helpful. I have decided that managers are self-centered. The road sweeper will give you more time than the bank manager.

I am much more trusting now. I need to talk to other people to find out their reaction to me. Once I didn't worry about anybody's reaction to me, now I do. That's a change.

Another change is that I live more for the present. Before, I used to know what was happening tomorrow. It was mapped out. Now it's vague. It's gone from 'I'll make them do this' to 'What will he make me do?'

Some of the services that I have used were better than others. The more services I used, the less resentful I felt about the help I was being offered.

I wanted to be as independent as possible. I had looked after myself since I was thirteen, and I didn't want to start being looked after. Even now I would prefer to cook dinner than to allow my daughter to do it. Neither of us enjoys each other's cooking. But that's another problem!

The workshop is boring, but it's better than being at home. It keeps my mind active to some degree, and it keeps me circulating. I think it's the service that's helped me most.

I look forward to Wednesdays, that's the day for the Fire Escape social group. There are people my age and with life experiences similar to mine there. I enjoy the social discourse, and the simple things like helping to make the coffee and tea.

The period of my life when I was introduced to the workshop and the Fire Escape is very vague. I remember that Fiona was involved, and I'm very grateful to her, but I don't remember details.

Red Cross has been invaluable. I have a going relationship with Barbara. We go shopping on Wednesday afternoons and I do enjoy it. The housekeeping and garden work that was provided before Meg came home was much appreciated.

Is there anything I'd do differently? No, I don't think there is. But I'm open to suggestions from anybody. How's that? *I am open to suggestions.*

Pauline and Cathy: A family under pressure

Pauline's story

During the two years prior to Rob's total collapse in October 1980, some strange events occurred.

Rob had retired from a high powered career in the advertising and sales promotion field to take on a new job as secretary in a real estate company. Somehow though, he could never make a complete break from his old firm, and he continually made contact with his former colleagues.

Rob began to work later more often, and we saw him at dinner once, or perhaps twice, during the week. It seemed out of character for him to keep saying, 'I sent so and so home as he looked tired,' or 'I told so and so to go early because he had a cold.' Suddenly, it seemed that he was doing his work and everyone else's work too.

The next really alarming thing was the development of a sudden and very real hatred for one of his fellow workers. This was quickly followed by an expressed hatred for his oldest and very dear friend of many years. This friend was a career diplomat and had not even been in Australia for almost three years. Here was something very wrong and not in any way logical, and I was really worried. I began at this stage to think Rob was working too hard and needed a holiday.

Not long after, Rob began to take a day off every so often and I had to phone his excuses. He would get up at the usual time, get the paper, have tea and then say, 'I've been ill all night. I'm going back to bed.' I knew very well that he had not been up during the night and had slept well.

One day off became two, then three, then a week with the same excuses. At this point, I began making appointments for Rob to see our GP, but they were always cancelled. I suggested retirement which was not at all well received. In fact, by this stage I refused to make any more calls on his behalf, saying, 'You want to stay home, you make your own calls.' I was frantic with worry: I knew I was getting nowhere, and I knew something was very wrong. I has this feeling that this was the beginning of something that was going to take over our lives and I was powerless to help.

Then came 5 October 1980. Rob did the normal things and left for the office at eight-thirty. At nine-thirty, the manager phoned to ask if Rob was at home, to which I replied, 'He had one call to make on the way to work, but he should be there by now.'

At eleven, there was a second call to say that Rob had gone to the office, taken one phone call, cleaned out his car and left the keys, then had walked out. Someone had seen him, walking towards the Yarra River.

Clutching at a last straw, I contacted my sister-in-law who lived in that area; but no, she had not seen him. By this stage, I was so afraid for his safety, and frantic. We called the police at three o'clock and they arrived to take details. Minutes later Rob walked in, not knowing where he had been, and in a state of complete limbo.

This was when we did get him to a doctor who offered marriage guidance, and Valium for Catherine and me. The doctor's diagnosis was marital problems, and a clean bill of health for Rob!

I was furious and wondering what I should do next. I knew full well there was something really wrong, but I hadn't any idea of what it could be.

There followed a period of his working frantically in the garden, as well as his wandering around town. And yet, I did not ever see him leave and he never could tell us where he had been or what he had done. I was very worried about his safety.

One morning, I woke to find Rob sitting on my bed alternately sobbing and babbling. Another trip to the doctor saw him admitted to the hospital where he was drugged until he was a zombie. After three weeks, I could see he was getting worse, heavily drugged, unable to stay still or communicate. It was on my authority that I brought Rob home and stopped all medication except for a sleeping pill.

We moved house for my sake as I couldn't cope with a big house and full-time nursing.

By this time, Rob was sitting in a chair just staring into space, between bouts of excessive wandering. He began to use the telephone: real estate firms to sell the new house, stockbroker, travel agents, bank manger, theater bookings, etc. So I had to unplug and hide the phone for the sake of our financial future.

I had gone through severe shock, extreme anger at doctors, bewilderment, loss of friends and the support of family. I wasn't eating, and was coping with my household with great difficulty.

I was so exhausted and frustrated. Then Cathy and I remembered how relaxed Rob had been on holiday in Vanuatu. We flew in and had two wonderful weeks; that was until Rob became agitated on the flight home and began to babble at the flight attendant.

We then asked to go on the public hospital system and were sent to Camberwell Clinic for tests. We were sent to a psychogeriatrician at the outpatients department of a major hospital where we were, finally, given a hearing. Tests, a CAT scan and the diagnosis, Alzheimer's disease. This was 1983.

After this I became more positive and thought about the retraining of stroke victims. I decided that, if I could get a spark of co-operation, I would see what I could do to get Rob doing something productive. That was the beginning of my one-to-one program of repetition and reward. It really worked for us, and Rob by 1985 was able to do most things. There were still flashes of anger, some vagueness, over-emotion and the inability to cope with any change in routine, or any unexpected situation. It was really as if I had an adult child in the house, but, on the whole, life was reasonable.

I think that my way of coping and the way I have coped must have some merit. In 1986, Rob's CAT scan had progressed from mild to moderate — yet his tests had improved from almost nil to between 4.5 and 8.5.

On a personal level, I know that I gave Rob my best for ten years, and that I did achieve something worthwhile. I have been through my personal Götterdämmerung and I'm still standing. I can understand why so many of my family turned away from the situation, but I often wonder if I shall every really forgive them for leaving the help and support to our sixteen-year-old daughter, Cathy.

Cathy's story

It's difficult to convey what it's like for a sixteen-year-old girl when her life is suddenly turned upside down. I had felt that all I could present would be a very biased view. But now, aged twenty-five, happily married with two beautiful daughters, I think I can look back to that time and give a fair view of it.

All of my life, as far back as I could remember, my parents had always been there for me. When Dad got sick, suddenly my happy teenage years were turned inside out.

My father whom I had idolised all my life had suddenly become short-tempered, forgetful and, on the whole, pretty impossible to live with. We attended counselling as a family to address the problem of coping with Dad's strange behaviour.

At our first counselling session, the doctor's answer to our problems was for us to take medication. I was sixteen-years-old, and the doctor was prescribing Valium for me! I didn't need sedatives, I needed someone to explain what had suddenly made our lives so unbearable.

What is that saying? 'Friends are there for life'? In my case, all my school friends, some of twelve years standing, had suddenly disappeared, afraid to come near our home.

In the years that were to follow, things went from bad to worse. I became more and more isolated from people my own age. I think I grew up very quickly during these years despite rarely leaving the house.

At the age of eighteen, I started to become friendly with some local people and began to enjoy life again. However, Dad was forever turning up and staying. Finally, my new friends just disappeared. They couldn't understand and didn't want a sixty-year-old man invading their lives.

I can't remember anyone ever admitting that there was anything wrong with Dad. It was all in our minds!

Work became my only outlet, as I'd become isolated again. Of course, I couldn't invite people home, because I never could be sure what Dad would do or say. I didn't bother associating with my workmates out of working hours.

Two years later, I moved from home into an apartment. I met my future husband, and slowly started to become a person my friends wanted to spend time with. During that year, I married, and, for the first time in a long while, began to feel that my life had become my own again. It has taken me a number of years to become a person that I can actually say I like.

I can now also say something that I had thought I would never say again: I am proud of my father for what he has achieved, and no longer have any resentment towards my family for the loss of my teenage years.

Les and Vera: A lot of tears under the shower

Les's story

When did I suspect that something was wrong? Well, I suppose the first signs were some years back when I was a foreman supervisor of a major transport group. I was supervising distributions at a chocolate cold store. We had to stock-take twice a week. There were a lot of problems there. I just couldn't understand why the figures would never jell. I didn't realise until years later that it was to do with my suffering from Alzheimer's disease.

It was only during my last job, delivering cordials, groceries, drinks and soft drinks and taking orders that it became really noticeable. I had a run to the next town, to a couple of hotels, three or four shops and a supermarket. The orders would be assembled a couple of days later. One of the lads said, 'Well, they have never had that stuff before.'

Of course, when someone went to do the delivery there, it was found that I was getting the names on the invoices of the orders crossed. Also, I was getting pretty bad-tempered. I think they just got fed up with me and gave me the sack.

I could never understand it. It was so frustrating because when I realised what I was doing, I made a real effort to stop it and figure out how I was doing it. But it still happened and I had no idea how. That really did break me up.

At one stage I went to see my doctor and said, 'Things are going wrong, and I can't understand what. Apart from not remembering things, simple everyday things, I put my glasses down and I can't find them and I go off to the lounge room or the kitchen to do something and I can't remember what I went there to do.'

He sort of brushed it off, and told me just to concentrate more. I tried, but it didn't work. I couldn't, for the life of me, remember. I knew there was something wrong, but I just didn't know what it was, what I was doing. I didn't understand any of it.

I finished up having a prostate operation. There was a woman there who came around just before the operation to do some test. She said, 'I want you to say these things after me and I want you to do some subtractions.'

One of the things I remember was subtracting from a hundred by sevens. I think I got to eighty something and I couldn't get any further.

I was having some problems with an infection after the operation, so I was constantly going back to the doctor and not getting anywhere.

I said, 'I don't understand what is happening. I keep doing things wrong all the time. I can't even go down the damn street now and get something without mucking it up.'

This was so frustrating. It just seemed ludicrous to keep telling a medical person that there was something wrong and not being able to explain what. I couldn't get it right in my head to talk to the man. He would ask the pertinent questions and I would answer them. It probably looked to him as if there was nothing wrong. Vera, my wife, was the only one who knew what was happening.

Vera and I went to a geriatrician. We were only there about twenty minutes. He just said straight out, 'Well, unfortunately, I think you have Alzheimer's disease. In fact, I am almost positive that you have it.' And that was that.

I don't think I understood the full implications of it then. In a sense, it was a relief because it labelled something mysterious, something I didn't understand. I went through all kinds of mixed-up feelings. Strange I guess, I was glad I knew what it was. That was something to work with.

I knew quite a bit about Alzheimer's. I remember when it first started appearing in the press, it interested me. I used to think it was an insidious thing. But when he told me I had it, I don't think I comprehended for quite a long time just what it meant, really, to me.

They had said, 'You might be all right for eight to ten years. But, of course, there is no way of knowing when it will finally happen or how bad you are going to get.'

I got very angry, especially when the man said that it is, or is thought to be, hereditary. I couldn't relate it to any of my family at all. That doesn't mean much. They don't discuss things like that. But I couldn't remember anybody with anything like it.

I went through much the same things as I have seen people with other serious illnesses go through. The reactions were all the same: angry, frustrated, confused. You want to hit back at something, but there is nothing there to hit back at. You don't understand why, why me?

We only had the one daughter with us and she didn't accept it. I don't know what Vera's reactions were because she never showed very much at all, oddly enough.

Vera took me to an Alzheimer's Society meeting. It was a support group addressed by two specialists from Melbourne. Everybody in the room was either a sister, nurse or carer. I don't think there were any sufferers there at all. They were instructing carers on what to do and how to do it. I couldn't get over the fact that I was there and nobody was talking about the patient. What about the person? What it means to the person has never, ever, been mentioned, anywhere I have been or by anyone I have spoken to.

Something has to be done about this attitude. Once you've got Alzheimer's, you're branded. That was terrible. It still is terrible. I can't come to grips with that at all. It is so frustrating. Because I have Alzheimer's, what I say is irrelevant: nobody will listen.

'He has got it all confused,' people often say. 'He doesn't know what he means, he's got it confused.'

I'd know damn well what I was saying. I wasn't confused. It was not a matter of wanting my point of view agreed with. It was wanting them to understand what I was saying. I know I did have, or probably still do have, a lot of difficulty in explaining things, but the basis of whatever I am talking about is there.

I was warned that I might find noise a problem at some time down the line. I always said that it had never worried me before, so I didn't see any reason why it should start then. Some time later, my family and I went to a club down the river for a big night out. It is only a small club, but the place was packed. The racket was just too much for me and I went and sat outside. It suddenly dawned on me: 'The bloody noise; I couldn't handle the noise. It never worried me before, why is it worrying me now? Is it because I've been told about it that I am aware of it now?'

There are some situations where I've actually bolted and got away from people because I couldn't handle it, everyone talking together. These days, I avoid noise as much as I can. I rarely go anywhere. I don't want to be caught in a situation that I can't handle or haven't got a way of getting out of.

The domestic scene has been very difficult for me. A year ago, I got into a pretty bad way. I didn't know what I was going to do next so I saw a counsellor at the Family Care Center. I had to talk to someone, because I was definitely going over the side. I desperately needed to get out at the time. I needed, I wanted, to run. I couldn't handle it. I had nowhere to go and no money to do it with. There was no insulting or anything like that at home. It was just a rotten atmosphere to live in. I was having trouble dealing with the Alzheimer's.

Most of the time I think I know when I am getting a bit confused. If I am left to my own devices I can take my time with something, and normally work it through. Things were pretty bad while visiting my family in Tasmania at one stage. Mom had to go into some type of environment where she could be looked after. We couldn't have her living at home alone because if she fell over, she'd have stayed down, she'd have been history. That was a very involved situation. I was dealing with allocation people from various government departments, trying to get a bed for Mom, trying to stress how severe her case was. That was a day and a half of absolute hell.

I wrote everything down. After each phone call, I would write it down, and usually by three o'clock it was finished for the day. I would sit down, I would read it all, work it through and say, 'Well, I haven't actually panicked. I haven't really stuffed it up, so that's OK for today.' It did happen once towards the end of it. Fortunately, there was a visiting nursing sister who called in and she got me out of it at the last minute.

Once when I landed at the airport and had to get the bus to my family's place, I discovered there were no buses. So, I was stranded at the airport. I thought, 'Well the only way I can get out of this is to get a taxi and go into town and catch the bus there,' which I did. So nothing really happened, although I felt uncomfortable.

Later, when my brother came from another state, he rang me the night before, and told me the time his flight got in. I didn't think to ask the flight number. He wasn't on a plane at the time he gave me. There was only one aircraft and he wasn't on it. I was in real strife and I sat there and bawled, because I didn't know what to do. My mother was up the road at the nursing home that I had just left. I was stuck. I had no idea what to do when, lo and behold, he stepped off the plane. You have no idea what a relief it was.

My brother doesn't understand much about it. He just knows that I am crook (not right) and he is sorry about it. He doesn't dwell on it and he doesn't allow it to worry him. I've got a younger brother and sister, both married. The sister is a widow with three teenage kids. They don't accept that I've got it. They think it is all in my mind. My sister-in-law said straight out in front of the young brother, 'He hasn't got Alzheimer's.'

'Oh!' I thought, 'I can't go through this again!'

I just said, 'Look, I can tell you some things that have happened. You work out what you think they are. I think it is Alzheimer's. Since I've been told it was Alzheimer's, I assume that's what it is.'

'Have you ever got a second opinion?'

'Why would I want a second opinion? Why would I want to do it? I don't doubt that the specialist was pretty right. He had no hesitation in putting it down.'

Mom found it hard to believe, although I think she accepted it.

I have two children from a previous marriage. My son says he finds it hard to believe because most of the time we have talked, I have been rational and he has seldom seen anything that he doubts. My daughter is more open about it. She thinks there is something wrong. She is not quite sure that it is Alzheimer's though. And she wonders if I should have had another opinion.

The perception people have of the disease is of highly confused, very sick people. I suppose I understand it better from nurses who have worked in institutions with really sick people. There is no way that I am going to live like that. I saw it at the day care center. I'm not going to be put in that environment. I'd shoot myself after what I'd seen going on here. There's nothing wrong with the people looking after them, they are trained people, and they've got this kennel full of pups, but everyone's an individual and everyone's different, but they are all treated the same. You all come out and you all stand there, you all have a cup of tea and now you all make party caps. That's not for me, I'm not that far gone. I should never have been in that environment, I should never have been made to look at what was going to happen to me. That was terrible and I have never been back since.

I didn't know it at the time, but it was really getting me down. To see what was going on around me at the day center was driving me down and down. They will tell you, too, that I wouldn't talk to anyone there. When I did, it was utter garbage, nothing would come out. It was a long time before I realised that the place itself was causing it. I am pretty proud of the fact that I recognised it and got the hell out of there.

I got away from everything and everybody. I wouldn't talk to anybody. If anyone came to the house, I usually went to my own room. If there was any more than one visitor, I wouldn't stay. I would make an excuse. It was obvious that I was not going to have anything worthwhile to say, as far as they were concerned.

We managed to scrape up the money to buy this farm and I often wondered if I did the right thing. There were so many things I wanted to do before I got crook. This was one of my main goals in life, to get my own farm.

When I was diagnosed, I thought I could still get the land and set it up for my wife and daughter. It would keep me occupied and that might prolong the process. Now I've found that since I returned from visiting my family, I've got straight back into a rut again. I've got no money to do the things that need to be done here yet. The worst of it is I don't get a pension any more with Vera working full-time. I understand that but the fact is that I don't have an income and that hurts a hell of a lot. Vera has to carry a lot on her own shoulders.

One experience showed me that there are warning signs of confusion coming on or situations that might cause confusion. Vera has a niece who lives in the next town, and the young husband has bought himself a truck. I went with him once and it turned out to be an absolutely disastrous trip.

It took us a week to get back home. We had two hours sleep on the way back. That was bad news for me. He wanted me to drive but I was too frightened of it. It was unusual considering the miles I have driven.

When we eventually got back, all I wanted was a shower and to lie down and relax. I got everything organised on my bed, clothes, everything ready to have a shower. But I couldn't figure out to take the clothes into the bathroom, or to have a shower and come back to the bedroom and get dressed or what to do. I sat there for a good ten or fifteen minutes and I couldn't get out of the bedroom. I called and frightened the poor niece.

'Just take your clothes and go and have a shower,' she said.

As soon as she said that, I was as good as gold. I just couldn't work it out, I couldn't do it. That frightened me. It was some time later that I realised that it had been a nightmare of a trip without much sleep. That might have been the cause.

Now, I look for warning signs. I look for situations I can find myself going into that I might not be able to handle. It doesn't always work because there are a lot of times when you are caught off guard. I think it is important not to dwell on it. You have to accept that there is nothing you can do. You can't have an operation to remove it like a tumour. All you can do is to keep doing what you normally do. Keep at it.

When I found areas that were a problem, my way out was to go and hide. I know they say running away doesn't solve anything, but in my particular case it did help. Some people might find that being on their own is worse. For me it is good. It's important not to let other people who think they're being helpful influence you. Stick up for your rights, you do it yourself. That is important I reckon.

In a discussion about something, if you find that people are not taking too much notice of what you are saying, walk away. You know in a flash what they are thinking, their attitude is a signal. A lot of people don't give you credit for having any faculties at all.

I think it is like living with a dying person. There are no answers, no easy way. You just have to accept it and get on with it and be aware of that person. It seems to me most people immediately are on their guard. They are confronted with a situation where they don't know the answers and they don't know what to do.

I worry about the future only in as much as I don't want to be messed around with. It is useless having an existence, a human body with no meaning in it. I would rather be put out in the back-room with the door shut. If what the doctor says is right, and you can live for years with the thing and still be a vegetable, you should be got rid of, because all you are doing is hurting a lot of people around you. I really believe that. I saw that at the day care center.

For the present, I just keep going the way I am. There is nothing I can do to change anything. I work. If we were financially sound, I would proceed to things I want to do: the draft horses, putting the block right, doing the various pieces of furniture I want to, making a really exquisite cactus garden. I would like to be able to do things like that. That and a lot of reading would keep my mind occupied. That's as far as I can go. I don't have any ambitions now. This is it. I suppose in a sense I was fortunate enough to be able to get this far.

Vera's story

My name is Vera. I am married to Les. For both of us it is our second marriage. Les was diagnosed as having Alzheimer's disease two years ago. We live on a small farm in the country.

The early signs of the disease were clear. That's easy to say in retrospect. It started with Les's inability to make up his mind about little things, like what he wanted to eat. That can just be food fads but this was too constant, total indecision. His withdrawal from initiating conversation was another sign. If it had been just with me, then I would have thought perhaps it was a personality thing or depression. But even when he was out, he would never be able to start a conversation.

His job had involved being a leader. I wrongly associated a lot of his withdrawal in the beginning with his losing jobs, and thought that it was just depression and loss of self-esteem. But when I look back now, I think it was far more than that. It was that he lost that ability, which is still impaired. It has recovered a bit but it takes him a long time to get around to doing something. But I'm amazed at the amount that he is able to do.

What is it like living with Les? How does Les make his decisions? Occasionally, he'll ask someone else for advice, or he uses people, especially me, as a sounding board. I try to take that role because I figure that's keeping him thinking about things. It's a lot better for his self-esteem and confidence if he works something out for himself. It takes skilled questioning and skilled conversation to be able to help him figure things out. I haven't found that difficult. Perhaps that comes from being a teacher. I had to learn how to use those skills.

I believe it is important to encourage his sense of his self-worth. There are lots and lots of times when he thinks he's done something that's right and I've slipped around behind him and fixed it up without his realising it. It's like being a shadow. The only time I'll intervene is if he's likely to do himself an injury. It sounds anti-feminist, as if I'm taking a minor role because I'm female, but I'm fairly strongly feminist. It's not about that. The person needs to have self-esteem and needs to have it built up. The basic things that you pick up in teacher training about self-esteem and confidence, work marvellously with Alzheimer's sufferers in the early stages. If you can keep them in that early stage and on that plateau as long as possible, that's going to keep them out of nursing homes so much longer.

I don't know what's going to happen when Les reaches the stage when he needs full-time supervision. At least I'll have enough time up my sleeve to take leave to be there full-time. Unfortunately I can't predict his behaviour. I've tried but as surely as I predict one way, he'll go an unpredictable way. The only thing I can forecast is his getting overtired.

I can tell when things are going particularly badly. Usually he sleeps in, withdraws and doesn't talk to me. His legs go.

'My legs won't operate properly,' he says, and he'll occasionally walk into a door.

If he gets the flu or a cold, he becomes withdrawn and confused. He goes very quiet, sitting and reading, unwilling to be out and about. A while back he was so erratic you wouldn't know what was going to happen next.

Les went through a stage of total rejection of any conversation between my daughter and any males of her age. She was seventeen, at school, making her debut, and she's quite attractive. Kids of that age just talk to one another without it having any particular meaning to it.

I knew he was in one of those moods one day when she was coming home. A boy she knew rode past, came back, and rode with her. It was very hot, so Les only had his underpants on. He got tangled up getting his shorts on, and I had enough time to get out in the street and warn them.

Aggression — physical, verbal and psychological, was a big problem for Les, one I found hard to deal with. We had to hide the gun, because we were a bit worried that he'd either take it to himself or he'd get too aggressive towards others.

It seemed to involve an exaggeration of his basic prejudices. If you look at his life as a child, and the fears and the prejudices he developed then, what you see now are those same prejudices just accentuated, without the social damper that he would normally put on them.

The problems with my daughter and the general aggressiveness are examples of how his inhibitions began to diminish. Sometimes he becomes totally uninhibited and totally unreasonable. Alzheimer's disease obviously strips away socialisation and social understanding.

Balancing the demands of the kids, my own need to survive, and Les's needs has not been easy. It is very, very difficult being the one in the middle. Before Les was diagnosed, I went to see a psychological counsellor, mainly because I couldn't get the two ends together. I got to that stage where I knew that things were going badly, but that I couldn't make them better.

At first I just tried to avoid the difficult situations. I'd tell myself: It's just patience, tolerance, understanding and a lot of tears under the shower. You've got to let it out. I still think it's valuable to let out your emotions, under the shower or to another person. The trouble is that there are not many doctors who understand and there are not many psychologists, especially in remote areas.

Les's personality change was hard to take, especially when he declared that he'd stopped loving me and moved to his own room. The physical relationship was one of the first things to go, but then he wouldn't even talk to me. He said there was nothing to say.

Looking back, it was really horrific. But you've got to think of it as being the disease and not the person. I found that if I could think of it as just a mask he was wearing it helped. I've even said to him at times, 'I don't really care what you say to me, I still love you.'

I had to find a part in myself where I kept loving him even if he didn't want me to. I keep what he used to be inside me and love that, rather than getting hurt by the Les who's there now. However, it's very difficult for teenage children to understand the vulnerability of the situation.

I'm not sure whether knowing formally that Les had Alzheimer's disease helped a lot. When he was actually diagnosed, it was more or less only a confirmation of what I'd figured out already. Actually, it was a relief to know it wasn't a major psychological problem, or that he wasn't heading for a mental breakdown. So, it probably was a relief in that way, but I think I'd known for a long time that there was a major physical problem.

I grieved a little at a time. Once it was actually out in the open, once the disease had been diagnosed, it came to reality. Rather than immediately starting to cope with the situation, I grieved for a long while for something that was dying in Les, even though that person was there. I cried quite a lot. It helps. It lets it all out. But once you've got the main grieving time over, you can start appreciating what time you have left with that person.

We were able to buy the property about this time, and that was very important. We could give Les a place where he would be secure and in which he could participate. We had to look for a place that I could manage, despite the snakes and mice. It's amazing what you learn to do! However, we had accepted that Les was going to be limited. It was a risk because it was likely that I was going to have to look after the place, produce an income, and look after Les all at once. But it has proved to be the best thing. He has peace and quiet and he has his own place that he can plan and develop. He more or less has a free hand to do whatever he wants, but he doesn't have the confidence yet.

Most of the people we come into contact with know that they can't accept a major decision from him alone, that it always has to be done by both of us. That way, I can take someone aside and say, 'Hold off for a while, because it's not what we really want.'

We are very fortunate because a lot of people up here know a reasonable amount about the disease. And, of course, in the country, word goes around very quickly. For example, watering our place is a bit difficult because it's not just a matter of turning on the tap. You've got to go quite a distance away and lift up a slide in the channel, let some water through, then go to another five different slides and do the same before the water actually gets to our place. The first time we did it, I was there. However, once Les tried it on his own. He didn't manipulate the slides very well, and almost flooded the goats out. There was water over the road. The previous owner who lives next door was good enough to come over, and quietly explained to Les what had gone wrong. He still comes to help if Les gets into diabolical trouble.

Les won't go to the shop now unless he's got the exact money because he can't work out the change. He knows where his failings are, when he is not thinking adequately enough, and he'll either ask someone, get me or someone else to come in with him, or he'll explain to the person that he doesn't understand. Very often I'll get a phone call that night saying, 'Les told me to ring you and explain about...' I can explain their answer to him, slowly.

I also have to act as a memory store. The trick is to explain things to him exactly the same way every time. I use almost exactly the same words. At school, if a child doesn't understand something, I'll explain it ten different ways and they'll eventually understand it. As soon as I come home, I have to switch off and explain something in precisely the same way each time. That way, it will eventually sink in.

Sometimes Les will stop me half-way through an explanation. I can see him process what I've already explained and then he'll ask me to finish. We've adjusted to this reasonably well. It's a bit difficult for me to stop saying some things in mid-track, because I know he's just a little bit off understanding it. I'm frightened that if I stop, he'll lose it. I've had to learn to remember where I'm up to and what I said the time before. When he's ready, he'll say, 'Now, tell me the rest.'

Sometimes processing time can take up to an hour. We'll talk about something and he'll go back to work or to his pottering around. Much later, he'll come back and say, 'Now, the rest of it.'

Most of the time, we try to make decisions jointly. I go through all the paperwork to see if a proposal is feasible. With any that are not, I allow plenty of time for cooling off. Sometimes I'll encourage Les in another direction that will avoid the problem of saying, 'We can't afford it,' or 'It's not what we want'. If I were just to put forward a decision, it would undermine his standing and his sense of himself. I avoid having confrontations because they are destructive and he can't deal with them in any way whatsoever.

Estate sales are quite an experience! Beforehand, we go off in our separate directions to have a look at everything. I usually manage to find the auctioneer and his assistants before Les. Without his seeing me, I say to them, 'My husband has Alzheimer's disease. Sometimes his decisions aren't terribly practical. I'll be with him all the time. If you see me shake my head, please don't acknowledge his bid.' It's sneaky! But I have to avoid his loss of face.

Les is still driving, very carefully and very safely and by and large, he's very good with the car. Recently, however, when visiting with his family, his son lent him his car. It had fancy tachometers and those sorts of things. They upset Les considerably because he couldn't understand them.

He's always been a keen newspaper reader. When the Alzheimer's disease started to progress, he would, at first, blame his eyes. Then the glasses were wrong because he couldn't understand what was written. Next it was the journalists, because 'They just don't write like they used to write. They take the whole article to tell you what they're trying to say.' But since the confusion when he drove his son's car, he's actually admitting his difficulty.

He said that he just could not understand, and that it was like looking at something written in a foreign language. He knew that, somewhere in his head, the ability to read was there, but he just couldn't get it out. He says this often. It's in his head somewhere, but he just can't get it out. Like something being on the tip of your tongue, but you can't quite say it. The episode with the car is the first time that he's admitted it, and that's only been since he's got more confidence in himself.

Being put on the pension was traumatic for Les, and this really pushed the Alzheimer's symptoms a bit further. When Les's condition was diagnosed, he was very concerned about being put on an invalid pension. I think he was trying to say that his life was over, and that he was no good to anybody for anything.

We tried to interest him in helping at the day center where he went for physiotherapy for a while, but it didn't work out. He just couldn't be around people who were almost the same, or be reminded of what he was likely to become.

He did start painting, and he became interested in cooking Chinese food. He still cooks a little, but it's mainly casseroles. Like the Chinese food, grills are getting too quick for him now. He hasn't got time to think about what he's going to do.

We have a microwave oven, which needs fixing but it won't be. I can survive without it, and it's too quick, too stressful, for Les for cooking and he would feel inadequate.

His painting has been a great saviour. He can take a break and go back to it. He's got wonderful natural talent, because he'd never taken paintbrush to canvas prior to getting sick. I was going to a local center where they have open access day-classes, to do some word processing and I discovered a painting class. Previously Les had seen a sunset on the television and said he'd love to paint it, so I thought there was a chance that it might help to fill in some time in the early stages of the disease. He was accepted by all those little old ladies and one man who took him under their wing. Unfortunately after their Christmas break he just never went back — a pity because he was doing exquisite work and activities develop his confidence and self-esteem.

Patients who hallucinate worry me; I can't seem to accept that part of their behaviour. I don't know what I'll do if Les starts to do that. I think I'm trying to prepare myself now by looking at his past and to see what influence that has had on him and his behaviour.

He's paranoid about institutions and being institutionalised. This may become difficult later on. It may be a choice of that, or one of Les's relatives coming to help look after him at our own place.

What are the things that have helped me get through so far?

Sometimes I think I should have been in the entertainment business because no matter how bad you feel, you've got to put on a performance. There is no point in letting everybody else know that you're miserable. I am not a very good public speaker or very good at initiating conversation. So it's very often a matter of taking a deep breath, gritting my teeth and saying, 'Well, no-one else is going to do it', and just bursting out.

I think being able to put yourself 'out of yourself' in that way, being able to categorise things, put them in pigeon holes, is part of it. All right, you feel really lousy, but you say to yourself, 'I'm going to cry about it later. At the moment, it's not appropriate.'

You need a vivid imagination, an ability to take yourself off into the most incredible fantasy lands when you can. It's using escapism for basic stress management. So, if you can't sleep at night because you're worried terribly about what's going to happen to everything else, you take yourself off to a fantasy land, and you're asleep in no time. It's really important to have that ability, when the time is appropriate, to withdraw into a place that's your own and that you can enjoy, even if it is only a mental world. No-one can take that away from you: it's there all the time and you know that when things are bad you can go back to that place if you want.

I get a break for myself in my teaching and I enjoy playing tennis. Les doesn't need full-time care, just to have someone around, and supervision.

I haven't relied closely on friends. During really hard times, I go to professional counsellors. I'm determined, pig-headed, arrogant, Les says. I can be very stubborn and not let anyone see what is behind the exterior. Underneath, the real personality, I'm fairly delicate and shy. So, I just put on the facade to get through. If you let your sufferer see that you are worried about things, they would worry even more about what you are worried about. And if you can laugh together about things, that makes it so much easier.

I try to guide Les, without him seeing that I'm guiding him, into things that he can achieve and that he can cope with. I try to be there as his gopher or assistant, as he sees me, putting the right piece of wood in the right place so he can pick it up easily, or nudging the right ten nails into the right place instead of his getting the wrong ones. Or asking dumb questions, dumb questions! This is the tactic, asking dumb questions.

So, if Les is about to do something and has the wrong implement or the wrong thing to do it with, I'll ask a question, such as, 'Do you use a hammer or a screwdriver to put a nail in?' and it will make him think twice about it sometimes.

Les was divorced some five or six years before I even met him. It was because of my encouragement that he has made contact with his children again. He seems to be getting on all right with them, too. They don't always recognise that he has anything wrong with him.

Generally, I encounter a lot of denial, and people will see it only as memory failure. They don't see it as an intellectual incapacity, or a loss of social conditioning and other learned practices. The cover-ups get a bit tedious.

Initially, one of my own daughters wouldn't accept the diagnosis and said that the difficulties that Les and I were having were purely my fault.

'It's just that you're imagining it Mom, you're misinterpreting. You're being paranoid!'

She and Les were getting on so well and I was being rejected. But, I got used to it, and would think to myself, 'Well, it's good they've got this time together.'

Les's symptoms, and the characteristics of his deterioration, have been very similar to those of stress. I don't know whether or not that's normal for people who have Alzheimer's at a young age, but other people have totally different symptoms — hallucination, aggression, major personality changes — yet retain mental function except for some forgetfulness.

Basically I've treated Les as if he were suffering from stress, and so far, so good. In addition, I suppose, I have tried to encourage him to recognise and deal with his illness.

In our support group, we've talked a lot about whether the sufferer should be told or not. One family didn't tell their wife/mother that she had Alzheimer's and she keeps wanting to know why she can't get better. She's gone through a stressful time which has made her deteriorate even further. I feel, generally, that people should be told, but I suppose that it depends on the stage of the disease when they are diagnosed. If it is early, they may be able to understand, and acquire some useful coping skills.

Robert: My mom, *Mick*

For the past nine years I have looked after my mother who has Alzheimer's Disease. In March 1989, she was moved to a special accommodation home, and then in June, to an excellent nursing home.

Looking after a person with this affliction is very stressful. Writing up some of the experiences has been a sort of catharsis, you might say.

The *nom de plume*, *Mick*, was Mother's family nickname — as a girl, she had auburn hair. *Ginger Mick* was a comic strip character of the time and also had red hair.

Living with Mick

A dementing person is quite unpredictable, and it is this unpredictability which is the principal cause of stress to the carer. There is no gratitude and the environment is almost totally negative. The carer solves one problem only to be confronted with another. Just as imagined in the battle of the Somme, every trench had to be won and *Mick* was quite unable to relinquish authority gracefully. Every little assistance in housekeeping was interpreted as a statement of her incompetence. If only Mick could have done as she was asked and have been co-operative!

When caring for a person with dementia one learns a lot about people who suffer from the condition, but much more about so-called *rational* relations, friends, and acquaintances of the sufferer.

The consequences of the affliction and psychological game playing cannot be easily separated. The worst aspect of the early years was coping with statements that it was the carer who was suffering from psychological problems and the sufferer who was behaving as a normal ageing person. These statements were made in ignorance and were convenient for the individual not wishing to face the issues involved.

The human race seems unable to cope with dementia, because unless individuals have experienced it first hand, they are unable to understand it. After all, it is funny unless you are involved. The ABC (Australian Broadcasting Company) was able to make a successful TV series about living with dementia.

In dealing with the process of dementing, it is necessary to allow the person with dementia to shed their skills gradually. To allow this, one has to turn a blind eye to deteriorating home cleanliness and the destruction of crockery, upholstery, carpets and the like.

Health

In her thirties, *Mick* had turns. These were witnessed by her young son who was ushered away by his grandma. Unlike the present, aged grandmothers were once looked after by their daughters. Grandmothers were very useful in the home. After a turn *Mick* would rest, and within twenty-four hours she would return to her normal duties. I never heard a satisfactory diagnosis of these turns which became infrequent and then disappeared. *Mick* took pheno-barbitone after the Second World War, and later went on to *Amytal*. She was possibly of a nervous disposition, was anxious and relied, in the late seventies, on *Serepax* allegedly for sleep problems. Stress was possibly the cause of this state. Otherwise, apart from a hysterectomy, *Mick* remained very healthy until about 1980.

About 1981, *Mick* started to become vague. She had two black-outs and falls which broke her wrist and hand respectively. During this period a good friend, an ex-Western Desert sister, looked after her and said that the blackouts were TIAs — transient ischemic attacks. My brother took her to a diagnostician who, after being side-tracked by epilepsy, put her on to *Dilantin*.

I bought her a dosette which was loaded with tablets to be taken in the prescribed sequence. The *Dilantin* bottle was left near the dosette and *Mick* would fill its every opening with tablets. This alerted me that all was not well. The *Dilantin* treatment proved ineffective and was discontinued. On some mornings, she was unable to get up and appeared 'stoned'. At about this time she was often aggressive and behaved strangely.

In desperation, in 1982, I consulted with my own GP. I had suspected *Mick* might be drinking. There was always plenty of liquor in the house. My GP said he would take a blood test and test for everything, including syphilis. The outcome: excessive enzyme in her liver, and platelets in her blood which indicated heavy consumption of alcohol. The GP also recommended *Normasan* rather than *Serapax*.

A search revealed hidden bottles of brandy, so her game was up. We had a family meeting and read the riot act. *Mick* denied the drinking and was suitably shocked by our accusations. All liquor was removed from the house and the drinking stopped.

As the dementia progressed it became necessary to administer her drugs, as she was so confused she would ad lib *Normasan*. This was not as destructive as *Serapax*. All behaviour modifying drugs were discontinued about 1983, as they were just adding to the confusion.

Throughout her dementia, *Mick* suffered some infections on her leg or in other areas. With these she would become more confused so the procedure was to hit the infection with antibiotics and rapidly clear up the problem. On one occasion, she was admitted to a rehabilitation hospital as she persisted in picking at the bandage around the infected leg. This had to be stopped as a leg ulcer could have resulted. It is necessary for a dementing person to be physically fit to make their management easier.

On 12 March 1989, *Mick* was taken from her home and placed in a special accommodation home. This was recommended by her GP who had attended to her in February for a urinary tract infection. Unfortunately, during this period she was living without daily supervision.

The move to the special accommodation home was stressful to her. She had lost her sheet anchor. In the early settling in period she was given behaviour modifying drugs. Sadly, once *Mick* entered the home, medical control was outside the carer's responsibility, and generally the medical profession ignores communications with relatives.

Later, *Mick* was moved to hostel accommodation. Rumour was that she behaved badly and inevitably, I discovered by accident that they were giving her *Mogadon* at night. Any drug of this ilk seemed to add to her confusion. Drugs are the soft option.

On 31 July, *Mick* had a fit. She was unconscious for about half an hour. The following night, she went walkabout. She chose a wet, dark and dirty night to escape. She was discovered in somebody's garden at ten o'clock, three quarters of a mile east of her hostel, without her glasses and with two black eyes. She looked like a drowned cat. She was returned to the hostel but remained confused for a few days. The fit was diagnosed as being of epileptic nature, so (surprise, surprise) they put her on to *Dilantin*.

These occurrences had devastated *Mick* and she deteriorated dramatically. A week after her fit, she was admitted to hospital with a urinary tract infection, and at long last, for proper testing — not medical guessing. They took her off all drugs except the treatment for the urinary tract infection. Even *Lanoxin* and her diuretic were discontinued, and lo and behold, a nurse advised that *Mick* had had two further TIAs. The nurse said they were quite common. Had the medicos got it right at last?

After being discharged from hospital, she was re-admitted to the hostel, but the urinary tract problems had not been entirely corrected. *Mick* needed reminding to go to the toilet. Because this required additional supervision outside the scope of hostel accommodation, *Mick* was admitted to the nursing home in the retirement complex. She has improved remarkably since and her urinary tract problems are under control.

The first catastrophic reaction

In the early stages of her dementia, *Mick* became careless with dish-washing. At this time, *Mick* started to buy large quantities of a detergent concentrate which took her fancy. Eight packets were found in one of the kitchen cupboards. However, *Mick* ignored the proportions of water to concentrate, so the product did not remove grease. In anger, I threw one of the plastic bottle packs to the floor. *Mick* was standing about two metres away with a table between us. The bottle ricocheted from the floor and flew low through the bottom pane of the glass door. A catastrophic reaction resulted. *Mick* then telephoned her relatives and friends and said that I had thrown the bottle at her. The relatives accepted her story without verifying it with me.

Some time later, I was directed to read the excellent book *The 36 Hour Day*. It was here that I came across the use of the psychologist's term 'a catastrophic reaction' to describe a tantrum. If possible, such reactions are to be avoided as they are difficult to handle and upset the afflicted.

Interpretation of the affliction

There is much to read about dementia, some glib as in the daily press, some well put together in small brochures, from carers societies. As I perceive it, as the affliction progresses, the higher centers of the brain are damaged and the policeman in our head is no longer in charge. Normal control, developed over the years, is absent, so uncontrolled behaviour results. The personality defects, so obvious in the affliction, were always there, but without the policeman they surface with distressing results.

The sufferers appear to have a tape-recorder, with an endless tape, installed in their heads. Sometimes, the tapes are changed. The tape indexes at appropriate or inappropriate times so one gets sensible or nonsensical answers and, of course, tiresome repetition.

Obsessions and hallucinations

Mick's obsession about leaving her home and entering an old folks home surfaced decades before her dementia. It was so strong one wonders if it were not providential! This obsession recurred at the appropriate times during her dementia, and like the boy who cried wolf, it eventually happened.

Another obsession, with her cat, which came into her life after her dementia, was almost too much to tolerate. Sometimes, in the early mornings, *Mick* would awaken me and announce that I or some other man had appeared at the end of her bed and removed her cat to the vet to have it put down or otherwise have it removed. The cat was often still inside the house.

She still asks after it, even though it was run over some nine months ago.

Mick was convinced that the fellow across the road had chickens and that he would kill the cat if it attacked his chickens. She started to lock herself into her bedroom at night with the cat. A catastrophic reaction would result when it had to be removed each morning.

One day when I was getting desperate with *Mick's* hallucination, I asked the fellow to come and explain to her that he had no chickens and no malice towards her cat. When this was explained to *Mick*, she replied, 'Who told you this rubbish about the threat to my kitten?'

I said, 'You have made these statements on several occasions.'

She denied these statements and said to me, 'You are mad!'

The fellow thought I *was* mad and barely speaks to me now!

One should not use rational thinking with an irrational person, but the confrontation with the neighbour worked. *Mick* forgot about this threat to her cat, but still locked it in her bedroom at night.

Mick's sister, Mollie, was another obsession. Everything from misplaced hot-water bottles, crockery or brooms I had allegedly given to Mollie. If I left early or should be away, it was because I was visiting Mollie to plan an overseas trip. There must have been strong sibling rivalry, jealousy or resentment, as Mollie was the elder sister who perhaps dominated *Mick* in her childhood.

Early in *Mick's* dementia, she became fascinated with all manner of debris dropped in the street. When she still shopped, she would pick up bits of wire, all sorts of plastic geegaws and drinking-straws, and leave these outside my quarters for my return home.

She assumed that they would be valuable in my workshop. This preoccupation with used drinking-straws still persists today.

In the last two years, she has saved all spent Lipton teabags and cardboard milk containers, believing that there was a prize or money for these objects. Of course, we used to collect aluminium milk-bottle tops and tea-packets in the old days, for discounted household goods.

Mick had hallucinations throughout her dementia, and no medication given to her intensified this mental state.

Restlessness and mutterings

Early in *Mick's* dementia, she was very restless. She could not sit and peacefully watch television without fiddling with the remote control, or sit through a two-course meal without getting up and pursuing another task. No amount of reassurance would stop this behaviour. Gradually, this restlessness became so frequent that it was ignored. Later in her affliction, she would move aimlessly in and out of the house.

Early in the morning while she was still in bed, I could hear quite audible chatter, invariably about Mollie and me plotting to put her into a home and planning a trip abroad. Frequently, sitting quietly in her chair for any length of time, she would mutter away inanely. Before she was placed into a special accommodation home, she would often walk around the garden and would murmur to herself about the fear of entering a home, her obsession about Mollie and the plotting for our next trip abroad.

The morning ritual

I believed that it was essential that *Mick* was up before my daily departure. As she was unable to give herself medication, it was necessary to administer her daily dose of pills. She was rarely asleep, but I would leave her in bed as long as possible, then ask her to come out and receive the dosage. She would put on her dressing gown and slippers and present herself at the desk where the tablets were kept. After taking her tablets, she would come out to the garage to see me off, and close the door and front gates. This ritual had gone on for years, but gradually as *Mick's* dementia progressed, she could not be relied upon always to lock the garage door.

On most mornings, *Mick* would ask the time and then say, 'No-one goes to work that early. You are going to Mollie's to plan your trip abroad with her.' No matter what explanation was made, *Mick* would persist almost daily with this obsession. The antagonism to Mollie continued to manifest itself in a number of issues.

Bathing

Throughout her life, *Mick* used to take a bath. Showers were taboo! Ritually, before her affliction set in, she bathed after getting breakfast and I had gone.

A few years into her dementia, I was at home and heard the bath-water running. It stopped and after a few minutes, or were they seconds, the water ran to waste. Had she got into the bath at all? How do you check your mother's bathing without creating a catastrophic reaction? After I had observed the sequence on a number of occasions, I challenged *Mick*. The inevitable umbrage followed and she insisted that she had indeed had a bath.

Eventually, from the body odour and a fungus-type rash under her breasts, it was apparent that *Mick* was not bathing herself. How long had she carried on with this pretence? We do not know.

With the pretence now exposed, the Royal District Nursing Service was called in, but only offered two days of bathing. They came at irregular times, and *Mick* was always dressed. She would say, 'I am dressed. I have had my bath.' Many times the nurse would leave without achieving her objective.

One dedicated nurse called Julie, who was committed to treating people with dementia, would come regularly and always achieved her aim. Once *Mick*, in a catastrophic reaction, pulled a knife on Julie. All objects which could cause bodily harm were then removed from *Mick's* quarters.

People with dementia like regularity and like to be handled by the same person. The Home Nursing Service changed both the visiting time and personnel and this was a problem until Julie took over. Of course, she was entitled to days off also. The bathing problem continued for a number of years, but bathing twice weekly proved adequate.

Laxatives

Early in the affliction, *Mick* began to complain that she was constipated, and one would find containers of laxatives in strange hidey-holes. Old people do have bowel problems, but how does a son verify if there is a problem or not? The solution was available. Just turn off the stop-cock feeding water to the cistern, so *Mick* could not flush the toilet after use.

This done and the issues checked daily, we discovered that there was not a problem.

Provisioning and cooking

In 1981, *Mick* would go shopping as she had always done and would bring back, for example, the wrong brand of bread. *Mick* was asked why she did not purchase brand X. She would reply that there was no stock. After this was repeated, it became clear *Mick* was unable to discriminate. This alerted me to the beginning of the affliction.

Mick would buy many cans of pepper and other items that would take her fancy. Over considerable time, her shopping expeditions became less regular, then spasmodic, and finally she forgot altogether and it was left to me. During the period of deterioration necessities which *Mick* forgot had to be bought to keep her larder full.

She would buy large quantities of meat from the same family butcher. For a number of years she had been one of a very loyal group of customers. Eventually, to keep waste in check, I asked the butcher to restrict *Mick's* purchases. He would tell her she didn't need any more of this or that, and she would be satisfied with this explanation. Only the family butcher and pharmacists have any personal interest in their customers now.

Mick was a great and generous cook but gradually from 1981 her cooking deteriorated. Cabbage would be put on at three for a six o'clock meal, and the cooking smell would be throughout the house, well circulated by the heating system in winter. Excessive salt would be added to the vegetables. Roasts would be swimming in rancid fat, and that old-fashioned vegetable greener, bicarb of soda, would also be added in excess.

At weekends, *Mick* would bring tea and biscuits to my den or workshop at afternoon tea-time or at any time that she thought appropriate. Because dementia sufferers need to feel useful, I played along with this until I realised that up to ten tea bags were in the pot. Eventually this strong dose of caffeine had to be refused.

Visitors and Christmas cards

Mick was a very generous and enthusiastic hostess. She enjoyed entertaining and with little notice, she would put on a Sunday tea. But friendship is interaction and as *Mick* forgot about her acquaintances, so they forgot about her. Her friends would telephone and sometimes she could not remember the caller. Many of her friends moved miles away or even out of state as they aged, to be near their daughters, and *Mick* could not recall most of them. In the latter years of her affliction, only her daughter and son called to take her to dinner, nominally weekend about, to give the carer some respite.

A particular disappointment was that only one grandchild visited occasionally in the early years of the disease. We should not expect too much from these grandchildren, as they are issues of the 'me too' generation. As *Mick* has not seen them for years, she does not know who they are! She does not recall people who have come into her life since the dementia started.

When dementia strikes, one learns about those people who are too shallow to cope with the condition. Is it the human ability to block out unpleasant happenings or is it our education system

which avoids teaching about such things? We should educate
people in the matter, as the affliction will increase in our ageing
population.

Mick received Christmas cards from friends. She kept every one
but would not reply to them. *Mick* has, until recently, had a good
hand and constructs sentences well. Early in her dementia, I used
to sit down around Christmas time to help her send out her cards,
but she stubbornly refused to write them. She said she would send
them when she was ready, and reminded me she was quite capable
of carrying out the task herself. A catastrophic reaction would
result, so this help had to stop.

Letters, bills and telephone

Some two years ago, I discovered that my letters were being
steamed opened. At first, I thought the envelopes were being
damaged by the post office. I then had reason to look through
Mick's wardrobe and found there a letter addressed to me with a
check inside.

A lock was fitted to the letterbox. *Mick* obviously was very
annoyed with this so she forced the letterbox door. The lock was
repaired and a further device fitted. *Mick's* next move was to wait
for the postman and take the letters directly. I wrote a polite letter
to the postmaster, and requested that the postman not give letters
to *Mick*, but this request was ignored. Very few people will help
in controlling the behaviour of a person with dementia.

One day, when I was home, I saw *Mick* asking a boy passing to
help her force the letterbox door. She would try every device from
carving knives to kitchen forks, to stab the mail and remove it
through the aperture. After many weeks she suddenly forgot all
about this frustration and in her last weeks at home, locking the
letterbox became unnecessary.

Many bills were addressed to *Mick* over the years, although I
had to attend to their payment. *Mick* would focus on a particular
bill and withhold it. For example, the newsagent often had to wait

for his money. Eventually, I decided to transfer the account to my name and the problem ceased.

Even though the medicos knew of *Mick's* condition, and were advised in writing of the procedures for payment, they insisted on addressing her accounts to her. *Mick* always hid medical accounts, perhaps because, given her obsession, she saw each trip to a specialist as another issue that may require her admission to hospital or removal from home.

Throughout her dementia, *Mick* was always suspicious of any incoming or outgoing calls. I had an extension phone, and from the early days, she would monitor all telephone calls. When I challenged her, through the connection, about why she was listening in, she would reply, 'I was just about to make an outside call.' She always thought I was talking about her.

Cleanliness

It has been said that the elderly tend not to see dirt. *Mick*, early in her affliction, gave up dusting the house. She became increasingly careless in her dishwashing and only vacuumed occasionally and did not move the furniture. She forgot to use detergent and used cold water for dishwashing. In general, she became sloppy with cleaning pots and pans, as she slipped into more careless behaviour. Inevitably, she soiled her clothes, but this was readily solved, as a friendly neighbour ran a dry cleaning business and so *Mick's* clothes were sent there frequently. With personal interest involved, the neighbour made special efforts to remove stubborn stains.

During the two years that the cleaning lady came twice a week to clean *Mick's* quarters, she would find on a number of occasions, cat urine on the kitchen bench. Instead of ignoring it, or cleaning it up, she would telephone her supervisor and advise of this extraordinary happening. The supervisor would in turn ring me in my office and complain. There was no solution which would keep *Mick* happy, and disposal of the cats would only create another problem for me.

There were four options—remove *Mick*, put the cats down, fire the cleaning lady, or forget about it and clean it up myself. The latter was adopted.

I perceived that *Mick* became frustrated, knowing somewhere in the depths of her mind that she should perform certain practised tasks, but somehow she could not. She took short cuts, which made matters worse. One of these short cuts was to carelessly hose out the porches rather than scrub the tiles or apply an appropriate cleaner.

Electrical appliances

People with dementia are great tinkerers. In the early stages, *Mick* left the electric stove on by operating the time-clock at the same time as the oven switch. The solution was to disconnect the time-clock and leave other controls intact. On one occasion, when the electricity bill was enormous, I jumped to the conclusion that the stove had been left on for hours. An immediate solution involved a time-clock and contacts which would permit the stove to be available only for three periods per day, at meal times. After the device was built and about to be installed, the electricity authority sent a letter to say that they had misread the meter.

As *Mick* moved deeper into her dementia, she started making milk coffee drinks and hot chocolate drinks. Frequently the milk boiled over and both the saucepans and radiant tube elements buckled.

Mick would interrupt the automatic cycles of the washing machine which resulted in poorly rinsed clothes and itchy underwear. The solution was to install a lock on the laundry door but this could almost produce a catastrophic reaction and heavy hammering on the door with cries of 'You are ruining the clothes!'

The ageing TV had failed on a couple of occasions. The estimate for repair was so high that I decided to replace the set. Any device always had to be replaced with an identical item as retraining was impossible. Shopping around showed that remote controlled TV sets had become very complex and would be unsuitable, so repair was the only option.

When *Mick's* small portable radio failed, I made the mistake of buying a new one, but she was unable to adapt to it, despite its simplicity of operation.

One of *Mick's* interests was flowers, and she often placed a bowl of them on top of the TV. Alarmingly, she would water these with any receptacle whatever. With a few thousand volts driving the tube, I decided to erect a sloping top to the TV, to prevent her placing flower vases on it, but she managed to forcibly remove this.

The electric kettles were a constant problem. Initially, a kettle, with a safety cut-out to eject the plug, was used with an identical backup kettle. To avoid retraining on a new device, I repaired each as necessary till eventually, spares became unavailable. A new simple kettle was purchased and training effected. The kettle had a red reset button and when this kettle finally failed and repair was impossible, another kettle was purchased almost identical to the original, except the reset button was white. *Mick* could not understand how to reset the white button, so I wrote a note to 'Press here' and fixed it above the button. *Mick* would not reset this white button at the outlet allocated to the kettle, but would move the kettle to another outlet and miraculously she could reset the white button. Of course both outlets were alive. You may say, 'Why not paint the button red?'

Mick had always had an electric blanket, but when she took hot water bottles to bed believing that they were a cure-all, this comforter had to be removed.

Keys and bank books

In the early years of dementia, *Mick* would frequently lose the keys to all internal and external doors of the house. She could not remember where she had hidden, or put them. I eventually had replica keys cut to ensure access. Dementia is great for locksmiths.

The two rear doors of the house were fitted with mortice locks and it is impossible to copy this sort of key. The keys were carefully tied to the door handles with a length of bricklayer's line, but *Mick* cut the line and removed the keys to hide them.

At about the same time, while *Mick* was still shopping and cooking, she started to lose her bank books and obtain new ones from the bank. One enterprising bank officer suggested that she leave the bank book at the bank and when she required money she would present herself to the counter and the accountant would give her the book. This effective solution worked till she demanded that the book be given to her. *Mick* would frequently frustrate very effective controls to help her.

About four years ago, enduring power of attorney was obtained by her daughter, who operated *Mick's* account and gave her money as necessary. So that *Mick* did not lose too much dignity, she retained her savings bank book, but the account was operated by her daughter through the teller machine. This left *Mick* still able to operate her account in the usual manner. She did not reconcile the account or observe that other monies had been removed.

Gardening and the blocked sewer

Mick's interest in flowers is still strong. She still arranges flowers well and maintained this activity before leaving her home. However, she developed strange habits in both watering and the planting of cuttings. If a patch of lawn died she would persist in watering the barren area. This activity made the area worse, and no amount of telling would stop this practice. She would persist in watering without a nozzle being attached to the hose and so compacted the garden areas. When a nozzle was fitted in an effort to control this bad watering practice, *Mick* just cut it off.

Mick would collect all manner of plant stalks and just push them into the ground, advising that they would sprout. One found as many as eight such stalks sticking out in circles like little fortifications. These used to appear all over the garden.

In late 1984, the sewer blocked. The blockage was located and exposed. The pipes had settled over time and the sockets had cracked. *Mick* was told that she should not use the sewer or drainage system. This was ignored, but when the connection had to be made, *Mick* had to be closed off from the kitchen and bathroom areas so water did not pass while the connection was made. *Mick* could not understand this, and persisted in trying to gain entry to the ablution areas. She put on a great act. She was told to go next door for her toilet, but she would not.

Home-help

In 1981, as *Mick's* ability to do her tasks deteriorated, a home-help was engaged to do housework twice a week. *Mick* resented this intrusion into her domain. She interpreted it as implying that she was no longer capable of cleaning the house. Of course, this was true. Most housewives would be very happy to have home-help, but not *Mick*.

After about two years of this practice, the home-help was discontinued. *Mick's* sullen manner and paranoid interpretations of the purpose of help in the home were too much to bear. All this, and the home-help did not come cheaply!

Useful information

The best text I have found on caring for someone with Alzheimer's or related diseases, is *The 36 Hour Day* by Mace and Rabins which I have already referred to. This book requires reading and re-reading to fully understand the implications of the affliction.

I also found that the superb British weekly *The New Scientist* produces interesting articles on dementia. These occasional articles clear up the claims about so-called important breakthroughs in Alzheimer's treatments, which the daily press invariably misreport.

You and Stress by Montgomery and Evans was a valuable guide to stress control. The Miller-Smith life style assessment inventory listed was carefully reviewed and items in the inventory which could be corrected were. This resulted in an immediate improvement.

Physician's Desk Reference is a valuable reference to ensure that the side-effects of medication are monitored. This publication is available from most bookstores.

Psychology for the carer

As the carer is working in a 'totally' negative situation, I think it is important that he or she become aware of their own psychological deterioration. This is often difficult to see.

I was looking after *Mick*, and at the same time, holding down a demanding job. I worked with a boss who suffered from what the psychologists call conditional self-esteem. This is the condition where the person only achieves self-esteem by condemning all those around him or her.

The combined pressure of work and *Mick's* behaviour put great stress on me. This resulted in a disturbed sleep pattern which eventually built up to a sleep deficit. One needs good sleep to clean up the mind's filing cabinet.

A visit to the doctor resulted in the inevitable prescription for tranquillisers. A few of these made the condition worse, so I stopped taking them. The disturbed sleep persisted, and after putting up with this for perhaps two or three years, I went to a clinical psychologist for three sessions for $270. As it turned out, it was money well spent.

The psychologist recommended the book on stress control, and after a thorough reading of the text and practising the advice, gradually a better sleep pattern emerged. I obtained an immediate improvement by limiting alcohol, caffeine and by adopting a rigorous exercise routine.

Psychological counselling should not be overlooked when the carer comes to the end of their tether and should be available for carers as a matter of course.

The special accommodation home

In 1989, *Mick* was admitted to a special accommodation home dedicated to patients with dementia. It was an attic style, weatherboard home, some sixty to seventy years old and located in a leafy suburb. Entry was gained by pressing a bell at the front gate. An attendant, or the owner, would come and undo a chain and unlock the padlock, and you would be admitted. It was intimidating!

Mick was placed into a tiny two-bed room with lino on the floor, and cheap plywood furniture. There was no bed-lamp or bedside table. The women shared a four-drawer dresser. There was a commode chair between the beds. This was the only seat available. There was little room for any of *Mick's* personal effects. She never knew the name of the inmate who shared her room. The room looked out on to a rough garden and a lawn. The papered ceiling was water-stained and the paper was coming off.

A few of *Mick's* family made up a photo-montage of themselves, presumably to give her some security and feeling of belonging. Unfortunately, it was placed on the wall against her bed, so it was too far away for her to see. People do not comprehend that dementia victims generally do not recognise those people who have come into their lives after the affliction has commenced. All those family photos are no substitute for frequent personal visits, and are largely irrelevant if the afflicted cannot recognise the objects in the photograph.

The special accommodation home had no room allocated for private conversation. Visitors were escorted into a hallway and sat on a shabby two-place sofa. When the weather was fine, we sat with *Mick* in the garden away from the other inmates.

With this type of sub-standard accommodation, I made every attempt to visit *Mick*. The owner made outbound telephone communication difficult for the inmates. The visitors entered directly from outside into the livingroom, where all the inmates sat around staring at commercial TV or listening to tapes. They ate in the same area. The home did have visiting musicians, and other craft people to try and stimulate the interest of the inmates.

I considered the place undignified, and expensive for what it offered. The owner accommodated only people with dementia, so he did offer a service for those so afflicted. However, pushing people together who are in various stages of the affliction is a convenient soft option but not good for those who are somewhere between rational and irrational thinking.

Mick was taken out most weekends, although this appeared to cause stress on her return. She enjoyed going out to visit her remaining old mates, going to the Botanical Gardens, or just eating out. She could not comprehend why she was not taken home. Eventually we worked out a scheme which seemed to make her less anxious.

The nursing home

I was determined that there must be a better solution than the special accommodation home. No stone was left unturned, including a proposed return to her home at considerable cost. *Mick* was alternating between lucid and irrational thinking. After an independent medical assessment her immediate family, together with her niece, were able to get her into hostel accommodation.

Mick's health deteriorated, and consequently she was admitted into a nursing home in the complex. Initially, she was placed in a private room with bathroom en suite and an excellent view. Later, because of an accommodation shortage, she was relocated in a twin bedroom. She had considerable difficulty in adjusting but now, as her condition deteriorates, she is less aware that she shares her room. My gratitude for the complex's charitable act in admitting her to the hostel can never be adequately expressed.

The nursing home is excellently run and residents are treated with dignity. I believe strongly that sufferers should be housed in both dignified and well-designed surroundings, and, more importantly, that the former carer can be comfortable with the home.

I visit regularly; it's important in reassuring *Mick*. I think regular visits also add to the self-esteem of the staff. These people

have a very irksome job, and I expect it is good for them to know
that others are aware of this.

Mick's future

As I said above, in the last few months *Mick* has slowly deteriorated. She has had at least two more transient ischemic attacks, one
of which was witnessed as she sat in her chair in the common room.
Each attack takes its toll, but I can see her fighting back with
renewed vigour to re-establish her authority. She is now regularly
incontinent.

About three weeks ago, she was taken to see her younger brother
who has a farm in the country and is very sympathetic towards her.
They must have had a good relationship in childhood. Such a
journey, a few months ago, would have been too stressful.

She is not very communicative, but recognises me. She never
wants me to leave.

Sinemet is being administered to control her frustrating Parkin-
sonian tremor, but unfortunately the medication has constipation
as a side-effect. Her obstinacy makes her unmanageable at bath
time, so they are also giving her *Tovlon* to modify her aggression.
She eats well, but is very thin and is frail. Never one to stay in bed,
she rises early and spends most of her day seated in the common
room. She seems adjusted to the company of others similarly
afflicted.

Mick appears to have forgotten about returning home. She asks
about her cat and her garden, and regularly asks to be taken to see
her younger brother. Occasionally, she says, 'I have no memory
at all now, and I used to have such a good memory.'

She is gradually declining with irregular ups and downs, but she
is not ready to give in yet. It must be the unflinching anglo-celtic
stock!

Conclusion

A year has passed since *Mick* entered the nursing home. The 36-hour days have now gone! I visit the nursing home four times a week. Visits vary from half an hour to two hours in length. I drive her occasionally to the country. This is far less stressful than coping daily with her unpredictable behaviour. It is always difficult to compare psychologically how I felt then with how I feel now, but there is no doubt that I am a whole lot better as I successfully climb out of the great abyss.

PART THREE

DRAWING THE THREADS TOGETHER

Issues for people facing
Alzheimer's disease

The stories in Part Two provide unique insights into the diversity of ways in which people are affected by the progressive dementias. In Part Three, we wish to draw together some common threads found throughout the stories. We also wish to identify some of the key issues facing people with Alzheimer's disease and related disorders, and those who care for them.

The improvements in living standards and in medical knowledge and technology in the twentieth century have significantly improved the general health and, consequently, the longevity of people in the Western world. The cruel irony of this advancement is that, as people live longer, current medical practice cannot cure, prevent or treat the major chronic illness of old age, Alzheimer's disease. It is still one of the great unknowns of modern medicine. Longevity has brought with it its own distinct set of problems.

The real impact and significance of the disease often remains hidden within the private lives and emotions of so many individuals. It has many effects on the sufferer. It disrupts life-long goals for retirement. It entails the frustration of not being able to deal with day-to-day tasks that have been second nature for many years, and the depression of not being able to stop this process and the insidious destruction of one's own personality. For carers, it is the loss of a partner, of someone with whom to share the good and the bad, of a parent, of the image of the loving and caring grandparent, of a companion, or the inability to resolve unfinished business with a partner or parent. It is this emotional loss, the end of a particular kind of relationship, that is often so devastating.

The most appropriate image or metaphor to describe the progress of the disease is that of a reversal of the growth process. If our early childhood is the process of development from birth to adulthood, then dementia can be characterised as the gradual reduction and loss of physical and cognitive capacity, a second infancy. The analogy is also apt for primary carers, in that their experience appears to be similar to the stresses and roles of parenthood.

Many carers say things similar to those that new mothers say: 'It's not possible to really understand until you're in the experience.'

Anne says of her mother: 'I found it very difficult changing roles with my parents. For Mom, I did the motherly household caring chores, but I also needed to make decisions for her, guide and direct her like a child, comfort her like a child.'

Meg, speaking of her father, John, puts it almost identically: 'The memory loss has made Dad very dependent, and I find myself more in the role of parent to him. In some senses, the roles have reversed completely: he is more like a child and I am the one who has to be autocratic.'

Whereas normal development involves the acquisition of skills and the growth of relationships, dementia involves the dismantling of relationships, the gradual loss of skills and abilities, and a stripping away of social and moral conditioning. The constant demands, the social isolation, the unpredictability of behaviour through the various stages are, for the carer, like those experienced by a parent except that the process is in reverse.

The early signs

Alzheimer's is subtle in its onset. So often the symptoms are put down to depression, mental illness or marital tensions.

Bert tells us: 'Our youngest daughter retreated to her room. She seemed to think that I was to blame for the emotional tension which was now creeping relentlessly into our home. "Family problems are due only to lack of understanding."'

Pauline had much the same sort of reaction from her doctor: '... we did get him to a doctor who offered marriage guidance, and *Valium* for Catherine and me. The doctor's diagnosis was marital problems, and a clean bill of health for Rob!'

The early symptoms of increasing forgetfulness, mood changes, personality changes can also so often be attributed to other factors: retirement, stress, or role changes. It is not easy to recognise them as part of the pattern of the disease at the time. Bert says of his wife, Joyce: 'I thought this was due to stress brought about by high blood pressure which had reduced her power of concentration.'

Indeed, only the continuation and development of these traits over a period of time are indicative of the disease. Perhaps only those close at hand have the right perspective. Les says: 'Vera, my wife, was the only one who knew what was happening. She recognised that something was desperately wrong. But, of course, nobody else would see it.'

At the same time, it is important to recognise that occasional forgetfulness is a normal part of old age.

Nonetheless, there are three distinct signs of the early stages of dementing diseases, and the pattern of their development is quite marked. Most of the stories in this collection highlight a growing awareness by the carers of one or more of these signs and most of the authors, with hindsight, are able to recognise the pattern, although they report that it was not so obvious while they were living through the process. The common signs are:

a increasing forgetfulness and confusion

b changes in personality characteristics that have been established for many years

c increasing difficulties with problem solving.

Looking for help, early information and advice

The nature of these changes and the subtlety of the onset of dementia produce particular problems in the early stages of the disease. It is not surprising that many of the contributors spoke of difficulties they had in searching for assistance to find an explanation for behaviour that concerned them.

Often, for the person developing the disease, there is a concern to protect themselves and their loved ones from their own failing abilities. They seek to hide the true extent of their impairment to spare others worry. Margaret has noticed this tendency frequently in her professional work: '... the person with dementia is so adept at hiding their dementia that other family members and professionals find it hard to believe that there is anything wrong with the person, and wonder why the carer is making such a fuss about the person's behaviour.'

On other occasions, people go to the doctor seeking assistance or acknowledgement of a problem, and are told 'nothing is wrong', or are given a sedative or tranquilliser.

As Les says: 'It just seems ludicrous to keep telling a medical person that there was something wrong and not being able to explain what. I couldn't get it right in my head to talk to the man

... He would ask the pertinent questions and I would answer them. It probably looked to him as if there was nothing wrong.'

Carers face similar problems in getting the information they consider important about how to manage the disease. Most often what they seek is a clear statement of the nature of the illness, and the likely process of its development, and direction towards services that will help them cope practically and emotionally with what lies ahead.

Unfortunately, the stories in this book point often to people needing to try time and time again to find doctors and other health professionals who can address their needs.

Not all medical services are experienced in the particular needs of dementia sufferers and their carers. There is no harm in shopping around. Obtaining good information, seeking clarification from one's doctor or other professionals, finding out the services that are available to assist at the earliest possible point appears to be a critical factor in the effectiveness with which people deal with the disease.

Bert says of the information he received from medical practitioners: 'I wish I had known earlier about how the deterioration of memory might affect the patient. For me, understanding had to come first. Then, there was acceptance and finally the ability to cope. I feel it would be the same for most people.'

One of the areas of concern mentioned again and again by writers in this book is the lack of accurate information to be had about the disease and about management strategies. So often, carers are well into dealing with the disease and experiencing particular difficulties before they are given or seek out more detailed information.

The emotional and relational changes, the environmental, legal and financial modifications required are not ones that can be finalised in a short period. Similarly, carers need time to begin to acquire information important for maintaining their own health and psychological well-being.

Contributors give another reason for wanting this type of information early: the lack of guidance about what is realistic and acceptable in terms of stress and work-load for a person caring for someone with dementia at home. Because the majority of people with dementia are fit and well, they often live for many years with the disease depending on their age at onset. Hence, it is critical for carers to be able to pace the work and stress-loads to preserve energies for difficult and demanding periods.

Ern summarises it well: '... not until two years later, when we saw a different doctor at our clinic, who asked, "What about Alzheimer's?" was the diagnosis made clear. I realise now this was two years lost in adjustment time for me and in finding methods of coping.'

On a personal level, for both those with the disease and those who care for them, it seems crucial that comprehensive and accurate information about the nature of the disease, management strategies for it, and likely emotional reactions to it is sought early in its course.

Planning for the future

Because of the subtlety of onset of the disease, the difficulties for both sufferer and carer in getting accurate information early, and a natural reluctance to recognise one's growing incapacities, people also often find it difficult to recognise or come to terms with the need for forward planning.

Throughout this collection, writers stress the need to balance up the practical demands of providing support and assistance for the person affected with the emotional adjustments required of each party.

People with the disease and their carers are so often told that there is nothing they can do, or just to try to get on with life. Judith tells of one such reaction: 'Along the way, my sister and I had both spoken to Mum's doctor, and said we were concerned at her actions and thought she was getting very forgetful. He brushed us off and said there was nothing wrong, just the normal progress for a woman of her age. She was seventy-nine at this time.'

Often, at the time of diagnosis or recognition, there is an emotional dumbness or denial. Often people are not encouraged or assisted to deal with the realities of the disease.

However, one of the key lessons from the stories is that there are many things to be done to address the practical and emotional adjustments required.

Given the average span of ten to fifteen years for the disease, long-term planning is essential. For the person with the disease, there is a need to plan to maximise function, and to put their affairs in order with dignity.

For the primary carer, there is a real need to understand the long-haul nature of their caring role. Very practical considerations must be taken into account as well.

As Judith would have it: 'I'm sure it would be easier to manage the practical, day-to-day tests of patience if there was any way to get rid of the emotional ties.' In the real order, it does not seem possible for people to partition their lives quite so nicely.

From our observations, those who cope best with the disease are those who plan their approach to two major areas of likely difficulty in a concerted manner. This is not to suggest that one can lay out the future, but that one has to predict the major issues and crisis points and plan for them in advance.

These distinguishable but obviously interrelated areas, and the skills needed to tackle them are:

a *practical management* — which requires a determined pragmatism to deal with the complexity of the condition as it develops day by day

b *emotional stability* — which depends on a capacity to adjust to the role and relationship changes associated with the disease.

Practical management of the condition
HONESTY IN DEALING WITH THE REALITY OF THE DISEASE

One of the constant questions that arises throughout the stories is whether to tell people that they have Alzheimer's disease or not.

For so many carers, this issue poses a real dilemma. Many carers wish to spare their loved one loss of self-esteem and dignity. They are worried about whether this information will lead to depression or make the person more difficult to live with.

Yet, as Les's story indicates so clearly, the person with the disease often understands their own declining capacities. Often as well, the person tries to hide their deficiencies, or tries to deny what is happening to them when they have difficulties in having their intentions understood.

But the evidence in the stories, and certainly in the editors' experiences, is that, in the early and middle stages of the disease at least, there is a level of insight in the person with the disease.

How frustrating to know that you are losing the capacity to do tasks which have required no mental effort in the past, while no-one else recognises or affirms your difficulties in the early stages.

There is an enormous amount of pain in coming to terms with Alzheimer's disease for both the person and their loved ones. It is this pain that often leads to an intricate pattern of denial with occasional recognition that something is wrong.

It is our clear belief that people should be told they have Alzheimer's disease when it is detected in its early stages. Further, honest and accurate information should be available and accessible for the person with Alzheimer's disease when they indicate that they are ready to receive it.

As pointed out above, for the person with Alzheimer's, comprehensive information is critical in assisting them to recognise that they are not going mad, in helping them to explain their behaviour to others. It is important in learning to adapt their own behaviour, and to accommodate that of their loved ones, in dealing with their memory loss.

Vera tells of the situation that arose in the family of a member of her support group: 'One family didn't tell their wife/mother that she had Alzheimer's and she keeps wanting to know why she can't get better. She's gone through a stressful time which has made her deteriorate even further.'

Part of the reactive depression so often associated with the disease has its roots in the sufferer's fear of not being able to address the changes associated with the disease in a consistent, practical and realistic manner.

Anne's mother, for example, displayed this complex interactive pattern of emotion: 'Mom's illness was characterised by fear and depression, and all the aggression that went with it.'

People need to be supported as they come to recognise the disease and its consequences. Possible strategies include those used by carers who contributed to this book. Literature on the disease can be left around; discussion about it is initiated with the person affected.

Honesty in dealing with the affected individual's concerns is critical. It appears important to recognise how the experience of the person with the disease and that of their primary carers is often negated by others, with the best intentions. If, for example, the person says, 'I think I'm getting forgetful!' the response is generally one of denial: 'No, you are doing just fine.' Generally, we do not respond with 'Do you really think that you are getting forgetful?'

Honesty is an essential component in dealing with Alzheimer's disease. People have the right to know what is happening to them even if they do so selectively. While, at the time of diagnosis or recognition, they may not wish to deal with the information, they will recognise their failing capacities and will inevitably need to try to explain this.

RELATIONSHIP TENSIONS

Another consistent motif among contributors is the tension that often develops between the person with the disease and their primary carers. Particularly prior to diagnosis, the changes in personality and increasing inability to deal with decision-making appears to create enormous anxiety, aggression and tension between the parties.

Anne tells us of some of the pressures that developed between her mother and father: 'Later again, Dad became the unknown aggressor, the assailant, there to 'steal Ken's things', and murder her. There were times when she would be tragically convinced he had struck her, others when she would furiously challenge and goad him to do so. Sometimes she struck him.'

A number of contributors indicated that they thought their loved one was having a mental breakdown or that they were having major marital tensions. Ern's wife '... even expressed concern about all those girls that I taught at Senior Technical College, especially if I came home later than usual.' The dementias' subtlety of onset makes it difficult for carers to understand behaviour that is quite out of character.

Vera tells of having to cope with Les's aggression: 'Aggression, physical, verbal and psychological, was a big problem for Les, one I found hard to deal with. We had to hide the gun, because we were a bit worried that he'd either take it to himself or he'd get too aggressive towards others.'

It appears that the level of severity of this relationship tension and the ability to understand and accept it significantly affects the quality of care the primary carer can offer and length of time during which they can care for the sufferer at home.

Part of being able to deal with relationship tensions is to be forewarned of their likely development.
It is important to have good information about likely personality changes and problem behaviours, so that the sufferer is not blamed for difficult behaviour.

Communication strategies which stress the abilities of
the person with dementia rather than the incapacities,
have to be learned.

DEMENTIA — A FAMILY AFFAIR

Common to many of the stories is the emphasis on the impact of
the disease on all the family, both immediate and extended. In
Pauline's situation, for example, the disease had a very different
impact on each of her children. However, the loss of a father figure
meant that each of the children was affected. Les and Vera's
daughters were both deeply affected as the disease developed.

Alzheimer's disease affects not just the sufferer and their primary carer, but other children, brothers, sisters, grandchildren,
friends and associates. In dealing with the issue, the whole family
unit, both nuclear and extended, must be considered. It seems
important to understand this family context and to deal with the
impact of the disease on the family unit as early as possible.

For so many of those who wrote for this book, the family unit,
in part at least, was the prime support network for the principal
carer. Judith speaks of her husband: 'I was lucky to have the
husband I did; he was so understanding and supportive at all times.'
Even for those for whom dealing with the family proved difficult,
the wish to have their support was very strong.

This is a critical point for families themselves, but also for social
policy. The well-being of the person with the disease and their
capacity to live in their own home is inseparably connected with
the maintenance of the physical and psychological well-being of
the carer. The major factor that led families whose stories are part
of this book to seek residential care for someone with dementia was
the poor health and exhaustion of the primary carer, more than the
sufferer's level of frailty.

If government policy is to encourage older people and people
with a disability to live at home as long as possible then greater
focus must be given to the family unit, and specifically to policies
and programs that support primary carers.

Very practical strategies need to be adopted to short-circuit possible family misunderstandings.

Family meetings, literature for grandchildren and explaining the disease to social networks like the church or social clubs are valuable exercises in themselves. They are also useful signals to a wider support group of possible future needs for more extensive support for the primary carer.

'WHAT'S WRONG WITH YOU?'

Not all negative reactions occur close to home. The nature of the onset of the disease is generally so subtle that it is only those who are very close to the person affected who can recognise the changes.

A common theme in the stories in this book is that more remote family, friends and associates do not recognise the changes.

Beth had a letter from her husband's relatives overseas '... written by the eldest brother-in-law, and telling me on behalf of the family, that I was a terrible person, a hypochondriac who was trying to poison their brother with all that medication, and who was trying to palm him off and shrug off my responsibility as a wife. I received another such abusive letter when I wrote and told the sisters that I had put their brother in care.'

The concerns and doubts of the partner or primary friend are often negated by the person with the disease or by family and friends. 'She seems fine. I can't understand what you are talking about.'

A friend of Beth's husband 'went to see him all right, but then I received a quiet, but abusive phone call, asking me why I had put his friend in that dreadful place, with all those sick old people? I explained a bit about the sickness, but he never went near the place again.'

A number of examples in the stories indicate that family and close friends saw the difficulties as personality changes or marital tensions. It must be recognised that often the behaviour is both, but that the underlying cause is Alzheimer's.

The nature of the disease is such that people's behaviour can vary from day to day. Social etiquette and skills are often retained longer than many other skills. People manage to react to the basic formalities of a conversation. 'Hello. How are you? The weather has been good,' says the person with dementia and this provides the appearance of capacity. The subtle changes which are the hallmarks of the early onset of the disease require constancy and time to detect.

Joan understood this latter point: '... Friends. At first, I had encouraged their visits and listened to their advice. He did seem to nod or shake his head at the right moments. It could not be total loss of memory. It was useless to tell them that Henk was just as willing to kiss the hand of any nurse or kitchen maid. Few had experienced the care of a dementia patient.'

It is important to recognise the carers' concerns and not to negate their experiences; practical support is often the best kind of recognition. Dementia is disturbing, and people not closely associated with its progress sometimes have difficulty coming to terms with it. Throughout the stories there was a constant theme of not being able to explain strange and uncharacteristic behaviour. So often the family or community's response is to avoid awkward behaviour.

Ignorance and fear are perhaps the greatest enemies for a community in dealing with this disease, and they need to be tackled directly. Accurate information about the disease and its progress is the best first step. Contributors to this book suggest that there is a need to be persistent and assertive in dealing with both explicit and implicit prejudice.

Be clear with distant relatives and friends and acquaintances about what the nature of the disease is, and what its likely consequences will be.

Provide information to people who perhaps do not understand at first. Most contributors are definite that while support is appreciated, interfering or misguided sympathy is not.

If people will not come to terms with the reality of the disease, be persistent in asking them to. Ultimately, if they will not, it seems best to seek out others who will.

FINANCE AND ADMINISTRATION

One particularly sensitive matter that contributors report needs careful consideration early in the disease is the management and administration of the sufferer's financial and legal affairs. It is not hard to see why it can so easily become part of family and relationship tensions. And yet, if this matter is not attended to it can become a recurrent source of friction.

Judith notes the problem as it affected her family: 'We ended up having to take over the payment of all her accounts as she would forget them or worse still, try to pay them twice.'

It is not only a matter of legal necessity with wills, enduring powers of attorney, and the like, if one is to avoid more convoluted processes at a later stage. Doing so is one of the ways in which the dignity and integrity of the sufferer is respected. Vera's approach to the difficulty illustrates how it is sometimes not so easy to balance the need for respect with the real problems encountered: 'Most of the time, we try to make decisions jointly. I go through all the paperwork to see if a proposal is feasible. Most of them are, some of them aren't feasible. With any that are not, I allow plenty of time for cooling off. Sometimes I'll encourage Les in another direction that will avoid the problem of saying, 'We can't afford it,' or 'It's not what I want'.

Legal and financial matters have to be dealt with at some stage, and are best dealt with while the person with dementia can still participate in the decision-making process.

FLEXIBLE TACTICS

Carers display a wealth of imagination in dealing with the practical problems that arise because of the unusual behaviour of dementia sufferers.

Some are designed simply to protect the person with dementia from being embarrassed by their own incapacities. Vera gives one example: 'We have a microwave oven, but it needs fixing and it's not getting fixed. I can survive without it, and it's too quick, too stressful, for Les for cooking and he would feel inadequate.'

Others are vital to ensuring the personal safety of the person with dementia. They vary in complexity from Anne's 'tricky lock on the door that [her mother] never mastered' to Robert's solution with the stove: '... the stove had been left on for hours. An immediate solution involved a time-clock and contacts which would permit the stove to be available only for three periods per day, at meal times.'

Still others are designed to relieve the carer of the added burden of having to fix things up later. Pauline found with Rob: 'He began to use the telephone: real estate firms to sell the new house, stockbroker, travel agents, bank manager, theater bookings etc. So I had to unplug and hide the phone for the sake of our financial future.'

And yet others require the collaboration of helpful associates. Robert used this ploy: '... to keep waste in check, I asked the butcher to restrict Mick's purchases. He would tell her she didn't need any more of this or that, and so she would be satisfied with this explanation.'

Bert, however, makes two very good points about the limitations of this approach to practical difficulties: 'Handy hints, practical solutions must be tried at the right time; to do so too soon makes the sufferer even more aware of their disability and can cause trauma ... Handy hints to aid the sufferer are simply a stop gap. Their use is restricted to a specific time during the deterioration of any activity.'

Practical solutions to the routine problems caused by disordered behaviour of the dementia sufferer are important parts of coping strategies adopted by carers. They serve to reduce the burden on the carer, and to protect the person with dementia.

Swapping notes with others' carers, through support groups and the like, is said to be helpful to carers.

It seems to be important to be flexible in one's approach, and not to see these strategies as a panacea for all the difficulties that are to be encountered.

THE HOME ENVIRONMENT

One important and major set of practical decisions which needs early planning is the actual living situation within which the person with dementia will be cared for. Some of the options canvassed have strong emotional repercussions.

Joan decided to move accommodation, and then began to see the implications: 'The contents of five rooms had to be dispersed. Heirlooms were allotted to young members of the family; relics from Holland to my stepdaughter. Selling our collected antiques caused heart wrenching decisions, but the money was needed.'

For Vera, Les's security and dignity, and her ability to manage were prime considerations and led to buying a new house and property: 'I could be sure we would be able to give Les a place where he would be secure and in which he could participate. We decided to move out of town and buy a small farm. We had to look for a place that I could manage.'

Vicinity to carers and support networks, as well as to community care facilities, was, for several contributors, a major item to be taken into account. Anne tells us: 'Dad had prepared a flat he owned there for them to live in, so that, when she needed care, she could be placed in the excellent and familiar geriatric hospital there.'

Other carers could accommodate the person with dementia with appropriate modifications to their current abode. Ern had to make his residence more secure to manage wandering: 'There were more episodes of wandering, until I built a set of driveway gates secured with a combination lock which frustrated her attempts to go and see Mom. Mom had died some twenty years ago. At least, the gates allowed me to relax a little.'

Whether to shift house, or to consider home modifications, and what steps are needed to ensure stability and security of accommodation, are major questions needing attention during early planning. Two factors regularly inform decision making in these areas:

a the safety, security and dignity of the person with dementia

b the easing of the practical load of the carer.

COMMUNITY HEALTH AND SUPPORT SERVICES

Governments have placed great store in recent years on the value of expanding home and community services to meet the needs of older and disabled people and their carers. A surprising thread throughout these stories is the low level of usage of community services by carers. Given the high level of physical exhaustion and stress experienced by people with responsibility for primary care, it is important to consider why such services are not used.

Part of the reason seems to lie in the nature of the services provided. Most domiciliary services provide practical domestic assistance with tasks such as cleaning, shopping and personal care.

However, until the latter stages of the disease, the individual and his/her carers generally do not need such support. They have lots of time to clean and prepare meals. What they lack is social company, someone to listen to their frustrations without being judgemental, a friend for companionship.

Another major reason relates to the view amongst many carers that 'I can cope. It's my responsibility' — a reluctance to share the responsibilities of care.

Anne was afraid of her parents' likely reaction if help was sought: 'Dad was unable to bring himself to use Home Help or Meals on Wheels. Mom continually maintained that she did all the housework. And the garden! We knew there would be outrage if a stranger came in to do her house, or cook her meals.'

Robert tells us that his mother also displayed such a reluctance, and goes on to explain why: '... a home-help was engaged to do housework twice a week. *Mick* resented this intrusion into her domain. It was interpreted by *Mick* as implying that she was no longer capable of cleaning the house.'

There seem to be three main reasons why carers and dementia sufferers themselves are reluctant to have the responsibilities of care shared:

a   a mentality that views seeking support as an admission of failure

b   a perception amongst many people that such services are 'welfare services', and hence are to be avoided

c   the lack of early information and advice about services that are available.

Sometimes, the services provided seem remarkably insensitive to the realities that carers are facing day by day. Robert's cleaning lady could not cope with the byproducts of his mother's need to be constantly with her cats: '... a cleaning lady would come twice a week to clean *Mick's* quarters. On a number of occasions she would find cat urine on the kitchen bench. Instead of ignoring it, or cleaning it up, she would telephone her supervisor and advise of this extraordinary happening. The supervisor would in turn ring me in my office, and complain.'

Finally, by the time some carers recognise that they need support, the person with dementia is often highly dependent and quite intensive levels of support are required because the carer is so exhausted. This level of support is just not available in community settings, especially to people who live in more remote areas.

There is no reason why carers could not be part of the process of changing this situation. Bert has tried: 'These days, I recognise more the need for help for myself. I have helped the local community services to train two specific home help people.'

In addition to facing up to the emotional impediments which hinder a realistic appraisal of the usefulness of community support services, there is no harm in tackling service providers and decision makers about making the services more responsive to the needs of dementia sufferers and their carers. Perhaps with supplementation, they could form part of long-term plans for the care of the person with dementia.

RESPITE

While it is true that most community support services were not extensively used or highly regarded by most contributors, it is abundantly clear that there was one form of service that was seen as very helpful to carers, namely respite services in the form of day care and family relief.

Ern came to see day care as a godsend: 'Also of great help were the breaks I had when Dorothy went to day care sessions. I must admit I felt reluctant about letting her go to day care at first. But when time passed and her condition deteriorated, I found it to be an answer to the long days when I got pretty desperate.'

Judith's account is similar: 'Those days [for Mom] at the center proved to be my lifesavers — some days I was so tired that I felt ready to give in, but after each break I was able to keep going.'

The same theme is continued in carers' accounts of the value of family relief and more long-term respite. Ern came to rely on such respite as the burden of care increased: 'After about three years, respite breaks of a month, twice a year, helped. This increased to three times a year as the pressure built up.'

Beth expresses regret about a time when respite was not available for her husband (and points to some of the Catch 22 elements of the service system): 'The psychogeriatric hospital would not accept him on family relief because he was only sixty-two, and they claimed that he didn't reside in their "catchment area"'.

The major impediment to the use of respite was the reluctance of people with dementia or their carers to admit that 'they were like the other people there'. Les says of his visits to a day center: 'There is no way known that I am going to live like that. I saw it at the day care center.'

Perhaps though, this is a phenomenon that occurs only at first contact. John starts from a fairly grudging acceptance of day care services: 'The workshop is boring, but it's better than being at home ... [it] is more congenial than the wharf but there's no cut and thrust.'

But he also admits that his opinion changed with contact: 'The more services I used, the less resentful I felt about the help I was being offered ... [the Day Center] keeps my mind active to some degree, and it keeps me circulating. I think it's the service that's helped me most ... I look forward to Wednesdays, that's the day for the social group. There are people my age and with life experiences similar to mine there. I enjoy the social discourse, and the simple things like helping to make the coffee and tea.'

Of the community services spoken about by those who wrote for this book, overwhelmingly the one reported as being most useful was respite care, both long-term care and day care. Some initial reluctance to use respite was common, but there are indications that people with dementia find it helpful once a pattern of use is established. There seems no doubt that it can be vital for carers as pressure mounts.

PERMANENT RESIDENTIAL CARE

Contributors who have had to make the decision make it clear that placing a loved one in a nursing home, hostel, or special accommodation home is one of the hardest decisions they have come to make. Anne's father found it very difficult: 'So great was my father's commitment to his role as carer that he found acceptance very hard. He couldn't separate his life from Mum's ...'

Beth's story illustrates that the pressure in the situation is not all internal: 'Some of our friends were with us all the way; others were uncertain, but accepted that I knew what I was doing. Still others thought that I was the worst in the world, but were not willing to walk in my shoes.'

The pressures are not always against finding residential care for a sufferer. Sometimes, a combination of the needs of the person with dementia and those of the carer coalesce to make it the only practicable choice. Ern describes such a situation: 'Finally, an opportunity arose for my wife's long-term care in a special purpose hostel for Alzheimer's sufferers. I only agreed to this after considerable pressure from family, doctors and the staff at the geriatric hospital ... The inevitable thoughts arose in this situation. "Could I have hung on a bit longer? Did I do the right thing?"'

Some carers are spared the pressure of decision by a natural sequence of events as were Joan and Henk.

Finding appropriate accommodation once the decision is made or it becomes inevitable can, in itself, prove a major difficulty.

There seems no doubt from the stories in this collection that being part of the service network from the early stages of the disease facilitates finding accommodation.

But pressure does not disappear once accommodation is found. After the intensity of care offered to a person with later stage dementia, some carers find the alternatives available not very satisfactory. First impressions are often devastating. Anne describes hers about the psychogeriatric hospital to which her mother was admitted: 'Crowded, full of chairs, full of dependent elderly women. My first impression was one of gloom and lifelessness. This was my mother's worst fear realised ... I guiltily suppressed the sick knot in my stomach and the tears I longed to let go. "Oh, Mom! How could we leave you here?"' Robert paints a similar scenario: ' There was little room for any of *Mick's* personal effects. She never knew the name of the inmate who shared her room. The room looked out onto a rough garden and a lawn. The papered ceiling was water stained and the paper was coming off.'

Ultimately, though, it seems to be the level of dedication of the staff, and the quality of care offered which determines how people evaluate the facility in the long-term. Anne, for example, continues: 'It didn't take us too long to see the life and love that was really in that ward ... There, under supervision, medications were found that helped her sleep at night ...'

Some concerns are alleviated with the passage of time and as the person with dementia adapts to the new environment. Anne's story concludes: 'It was three months before Mom settled. Then, abruptly, fear left her. It seemed as though she realised she no longer had to prove anything, to pretend. She could just be ... and she adapted to the routine.'

Robert noticed the same acclimatisation with his mother: 'She seems adjusted to the company of others similarly afflicted. *Mick* appears to have forgotten about returning home. She asks about her cat and her garden, and regularly asks to be taken to see her younger brother.'

Provided that satisfactory care is, in fact, found, carers too acclimatise. In many cases, they feel relieved of a great burden and are able to enjoy once more their contact with the person they love, more than was possible in the final, very difficult stages of care at home. They begin to reconstruct their own lives, with new insight, and often with a great sense of pride. Robert expresses these sentiments: 'This is far less stressful than coping daily with her unpredictable behaviour. It is always difficult to compare psychologically how I felt then with how I feel now, but there is no doubt that I am a whole lot better as I successfully climb out of the great abyss.'

The period immediately following the admission of a person with dementia to residential care is often emotionally charged and difficult, both for the person with dementia and their former primary carer. If the quality of the residential care is satisfactory and staff are caring, both adjust with time. The final outcome is frequently much better for both than the final, very difficult stages of home care.

Emotional realities

THE DIFFERENT NEEDS OF PEOPLE WITH DEMENTIA AND THEIR PRIMARY CARERS

While considerable attention has been given to the emotional and lifestyle changes required by carers, minimal attention has been given to the type of information and assistance required by the person with the disease. In the past, this group have not come to public attention until their dementia is quite well developed. Their needs have, commonly, been represented by their primary care giver. Stigma, ignorance, isolation, lack of opportunity are all contributory factors. However, what must be recognised is that the needs of the person with the disease and their carers are not necessarily compatible. Different strategies may be required for each group.

For the person with dementia, it is critical to support them in dealing with the reality of their declining cognitive abilities. Recognition and acceptance of the reality of the disease is essential. Strategies such as group work, individual counselling, understanding the nature of their dementia and providing support through the reactions of family, friends and associates is essential. Respect for their dignity, shown in respect for their legal and financial preferences as well as those for treatment or care, is essential, and all the more so while the person still has the insight and legal capacity to express his/her wishes.

For the primary carer, there is a different set of life-issues to be addressed. While the person with the disease is struggling to come to terms with their loss of memory, the carer is trying to deal with the gradual loss of a partner or parent, negative feelings towards the person which may be generated through the onset of the disease, emotional adjustments to taking the 'lead role' in the relationship, and stressful practical changes to lifestyle.

Carers are deciding whether to stop work or try to balance the demands of work and home care. There is much work to be done organising the practical management of the care of their loved one: finding out information, understanding what services are available and the costs of assistance in the task of caring.

While a certain amount of this will be done together, the needs of each of the parties are distinctive. The differing nature of the needs of people with the disease and their carers should be recognised.

Getting the balance right is not easy. As Vera puts it: 'Balancing the demands of the kids, my own need to survive, and Les's needs has not been easy. It is very, very difficult being the one in the middle.'

Several of the contributors to this book reported not getting the balance right, usually at the expense of the carer. Ern tells the story: 'A relative in her late seventies and with poor health herself, battled on caring for her husband. He had had several small strokes and other health problems and didn't seem to notice what was being done for him or at what cost until she entered a hospital and died within two weeks.'

It is important to emphasise that the emotional needs of both people with dementia *and* those who care for them have to be considered.

The main predictor of the extent to which a carer will cope over the long-term is their ability to maintain good physical and emotional well-being. Burnout is a very real danger for carers and is often a counterproductive result of an intense desire to offer loyal support.

DEALING WITH THE NEGATIVES

One of the dominant negative emotions experienced by those who suffer from one of the dementias is fear. The fear of losing one's mental capacities is one of the major fears of people old and young. Recent publicity and awareness about the disease has highlighted concerns, particularly among older people, that they may be losing their minds.

Similarly, sufferers fear loss of control. Barbara has noted it in many of the people she has cared for: 'None of us enjoys being organised and pushed around faster than we can personally manage and not one of us likes to feel that we do not have control over our own lives.'

Fear needs to be named so that others can respond honestly. So often subjects which raise fears are not broached lest other people are upset or offended. More often, however, people are distressed by not being able to offer a loved one the care and support which makes fears tolerable.

Fear is most often of the unknown or unexpected. John, who saw his control dwindling and expressed some apprehension, takes a very practical approach to handling his fear: 'Another change is that I live more for the present. Before, I used to know what was happening tomorrow. It was mapped out. Now it's vague.'

Caring for someone at home has been described in the literature in terms of the title of the book *The 36 Hour Day* (Mace, 1983). Particularly in the second and third stages of the dementing diseases, it is a constant and frustrating task.

For the primary carer, the adjustments are many. In a number of ways, as the disease progresses, it is like adjusting to the needs of a demanding child. Carers can feel lots of anger and frustration, emotions which people learn to deal with differently depending on their life history.

Sometimes, these feelings are released verbally, emotionally or even physically on the person with the dementia.

Others bottle things up more, like Beth: 'I am sure that we were never made to keep our emotions under control to that degree. The pressure generated began to affect my health.' There are sometimes high levels of guilt about their negative attitudes or behaviour towards their loved one.

Many carers find it difficult to express these negative feelings to themselves let alone to their family and friends or outsiders.

Fear of loss of dignity, and ultimately of control and personality weigh heavily on the person with dementia. This is often accompanied by frustration at their inability to communicate effectively and to be taken seriously as a person with their own sensitivities and aspirations. Like carers, people with dementia grieve for opporunities denied and experiences curtailed. Beth reflects: 'My husband was too early with his illness'.

While it would be simplistic to assume that concentration on positive aspects of new relationships would solve all problems, some attempt to shift focus would seem helpful. Perhaps even a bit of humour. Anne speaks of it in her attempts to deal with her feelings about her mother: 'We soon began to highlight the humour, the absurd, and often our helpless laughter saved an otherwise unbearable situation'.

It seems important to reiterate what has become almost a truism in modern psychological writing: there is nothing wrong with negative feelings. It's all right to have them and it's all right to express them without doing violence to others. Often, this acknowledgement and expression is a vital part of the process of dealing with them constructively. One of the major advantages of support groups, for example, is that they provide the opportunity to express feelings in an environment in which people will understand and accept.

Negative feelings are part of the information we have available to us when we're making responsible decisions: they don't control what we do. They need to be balanced against more positive feelings which sometimes get lost in moments of stress: joyful memories, commitment, love and affection.

DIGNITY AND RESPECT

The clearest need for those who suffer from one of the dementias is to be able to maintain their dignity, respect and self-esteem. For John, this meant remaining independent for as long as he could: 'I wanted to be as independent as possible. I had looked after myself since I was thirteen, and I didn't want to start being looked after.'

The very nature of the disease whittles away independence. Barbara, after stressing the need to modify tasks to the capabilities of the person with dementia rather than the other way around, observes: 'Constant failure to complete tasks which are no longer possible, then, affects self-esteem, confidence and competence'. Meg notes one of the consequences of her father's dementia, but reinforces how important it is to encourage people with dementia to achieve what they can: 'He is reluctant to try new things, but actually enjoys them once he can be coaxed into doing it'.

Some of the factors which tend to diminish the dignity and self-esteem of people with dementia come from the social circumstances they encounter. One common reaction to people with dementia is to think they are mad. Beth tells of friends 'standing back from this terrible mysterious mental illness'.

Prejudices about mental illness exist deep in the human psyche and we are becoming more aware of how they operate to the disadvantage of people with psychiatric illnesses. They directly impinge on people with dementia. Dementia does involve socially awkward and, at times, difficult behaviours. People with the disease have difficulties communicating and they confuse concepts. They are often less inhibited. *But they are not mad.*

They often have some insight into the nature of their diseases. Barbara has observed this: 'For a long time, many people with Alzheimer's have a great deal of insight into their loss of memory, their muddlement, their making more and more errors, their inability to do adequately things that they have done with ease all their lives'.

Les has experienced the consequences that go with the diagnosis: 'Once you've got Alzheimer's, you're branded. That was terrible. It still is terrible. I can't come to grips with that at all. It is so frustrating. Because I've Alzheimer's, what I say is irrelevant: nobody will listen.'

Even the system designed to make their care easier is not free from fault and sometimes mitigates against people with dementia being accorded dignity and respect. Beth mentions the way their environments are made to change too often: 'Does anyone realise how hard it is for a confused person to learn a new environment? When is the system going to look at these patients as people, not pawns that have to be moved from one situation to another.'

People with dementia need support and assistance, but of a kind which respects their human dignity. The community has to adapt its understanding and skills and offer assistance which does this. Fear and stigma will only reinforce their isolation and result in higher levels of institutionalisation. The understanding and adjustments required are essential, and both sufferers and carers should have no hesitation in asserting themselves and their rights in the face of people or organisations who treat them with anything other than respect.

How is this done? Many people have great difficulty being *assertive*. Assertiveness is often mistaken for aggression. People who behave with aggression find in the long run that it is not really helpful in most situations because it does not accord to the other person the very respect it seeks. Rather, it seeks to express our needs and wishes at the expense of others. Further, it often escalates aggressive responses.

The same mistake leads other people to withdraw. They think being assertive is nothing other than being aggressive, and because they feel bad about being aggressive, they are passive, that is, they take no steps to ensure their feelings and thoughts are respected.

Assertive communication and behaviour, which is important for people seeking to establish that they should be treated with dignity and respect, takes place between people when there is an honest and open exchange of thoughts and feelings in a way that is socially acceptable and which respects the well-being and feelings of each person.

People who behave assertively display four major skills:

a   Their *body language* encourages the other person to take their thoughts and feelings seriously as they do themselves. Hence, they look directly at the other person when they speak. Their posture is open and direct: they face the other person, get close enough and hold their head erect. Their gestures and facial expressions reflect the content of what they have to say.

b   They use the *tone and volume of their voice* to reinforce their message. They do not shout or whisper, but speak in a cool, level voice geared at communicating rather than provoking a response.

c   They pick the *right time and place to deliver their message*. They do not embarrass people socially, or try to talk seriously and calmly when another is busy or in the heat of an argument, for example.

d   *The content of what they say* is a clear statement of the thoughts and feelings they have identified moderated against a concern to respect the other person. There are four components of a communication that is assertive in content:

   i)   it begins with an acknowledgement of the feelings of the other, and is careful not to back them into an emotional corner

   ii) it relies on the person making the communication identifying and owning their own thoughts and feelings

   iii) without blame, it points to the circumstances or situation in which the thoughts and feelings arise

   iv) it is the *minimum effective response*, or in other words, it achieves its goal by expressing the least amount of negative emotion necessary.

An example will illustrate the last point about content. Many of the contributors reported not being taken seriously when they first approached a professional about their problem. Nonetheless, they knew that there was a problem, and often felt frustrated and angry with the response they received. An assertive response to this set of circumstances would go something like this:

'Doctor, thank you for your time. I do appreciate that you are concerned not to cause us undue worry.

An acknowledgement of the genuine care and concern of the other person.

However, I am very frustrated because I know that there is something wrong even if I am having difficulty in explaining what it is to you.

A clear statement of what you feel, how strongly you feel it and why. Not blaming another person for your feelings, but owning them.

I would like a clear diagnosis of what the problem is, and further referral if you feel that you have done all you can.'

A clear statement of your needs which recognises the concerns and needs of the other person.

GUILT

Most carers who contributed to this book report being hit by guilt at one stage or another of the decision-making process associated with the disease. Anne experienced it when she took her mother to full-time residential care: 'Under a grateful facade, I guiltily suppressed the sick knot in my stomach and the tears I longed to let go. "Oh Mom! How could we leave you here?"' As did her father: 'He grieved bitterly, isolating himself, unable to let go of his guilt at his perceived failure as a caring husband.'

Judith experienced guilt because her decision, like most major decisions, was not cut and dried: 'I really didn't feel guilty with the decision to place Mom in a nursing home, rather, perhaps there was the guilt of feeling so relieved that the burden had been taken from us.'

Joan remembers her feeling about Henk going to a nursing home: 'But I do remember sobbing for most of the night — and accusing myself over and over.'

At the same time, none of the carers who reports feelings of guilt suggests practical strategies for dealing with it when it occurs. Some rely on the fact that time itself often heals feelings of guilt. Anne tells us her story: 'Only gradually has he [her father] come to a point, during the last year, when he could take up his own life and live beyond the hospital, participating again in his old activities and pleasures without feeling he is abandoning Mom.'

And for others, a decision that has only one aspect when it is made acquires others as new patterns come to light. Judith's story shows that even situations which seem to have an overwhelming downside can change as time throws its light on them: 'I began to feel so good in myself. I made up my mind to go back to work part-time and get my life back together again. I felt that the last two years were a phase that cannot be forgotten but also a time for me to dwell on. I felt again so much love for Mom. I didn't have that constant concern I felt near the end of the time she was with us, that my love was turning to resentment.'

But there are strategies for dealing with guilt. None of them can guarantee to take the feeling away but they do help to relieve the intensity of guilt feelings, and to allow us to proceed with good decision making.

How do you handle guilt feelings? First, *attack guilt intellectually*. The argument runs something like this:

Whatever its advantages in stopping children doing dangerous things while their mothers or fathers are not supervising them, guilt is not a helpful emotion for adults

trying to make decisions. It gets in the way of making good decisions for three reasons:

a   *Guilt has no sense of proportion.* You can feel extremely guilty about things that have no real moral weight, and yet be oblivious of things that are very important. The best example, a bit unconventional but useful if only because most people know the experience, is the way people feel absolutely terrible if caught picking their nose in the car at the traffic light. While the activity may seem a little unhygenic, most of us would acknowledge that it has little moral significance and is a matter of politeness. On the other hand, it is easy to have no guilt feelings at all about living in luxury while people in other parts of the world starve.

b   *Guilt has no sense of direction.* Many choices are not yes/no decisions. They involve the complex weighing of a whole set of alternatives. Guilt feelings may be able to deter us from doing this or that, but they focus on the past and do not point us to the best decision for the future.

c   *Guilt is transient.* It has no staying power for the long haul, and many of the decisions being made by dementia sufferers and their carers need a stronger base than that to see them through both good and bad times that lie ahead.

Secondly, *acknowledge your feelings of guilt.* Share them with others if it helps. There is nothing wrong with feeling guilty. There is a problem when guilt paralyses us and becomes a hidden agenda impeding responsible choices. Joan felt she had made the wrong decision in consenting too easily to her husband's surgery which marked the beginning of his severe dementia: 'The shock of four years ago had caused a kaleidoscope of emotions, the worst of which was guilt.'

Thirdly, *proceed to make your decisions anyway.* Seek good information; often knowledge is enough to relieve guilt on its own. This is what happened to Joan: 'His [the doctor's] advice, that multiple infarct dementia had been identified as a disease only in 1974, had finally extinguished my feelings of guilt.'

Make your decisions in a systematic way. Give yourself as much time as you can: better decisions are made when a time of immediate crisis has past. After getting accurate information, look at the whole network of relationships of which you are part. Consider the *long-term* impact of your decision on *yourself,* and on *all* the people who are important to you. Jot down the gains and losses if it helps. Consult people who are part of your network if you are not sure about the impact. Swap ideas with people who are a little more detached from the situation.

Finally, *take decisions which expand rather than constrict your options.* This involves a willingness to revise options and to admit mistakes. If a mistake is made, the process can begin again.

Do anything else you like, but adamantly refuse to feel guilty. Particularly, do not let guilt stand in the way of taking a stand which is in the long-term best interests of yourself and your relationships with the broad range of people you are close to.

STRESS

Stress is not necessarily a bad thing; it is part of the natural way our bodies gear up to face a challenge. But too much stress can detract from our general capacity to cope, and there is not doubt that dementia puts firstly both sufferer and carer, and ultimately mainly the carer, under an inordinate degree of stress.

Margaret noted its impact consistently in her professional work: 'I was always acutely aware of the high levels of stress experienced by carers in trying to come to terms with the disease, and as the result of their caring role.'

Robert reports experiencing some of the symptoms of undue stress: 'The combined pressure of work and *Mick's* behaviour put great stress on me. This resulted in a disturbed sleep pattern which eventually built up to a sleep deficit. One needs good sleep to clean up the mind's filing cabinet.'

Pauline also found that the level of stress affected her physically: 'I wasn't eating, and was coping with my household with great difficulty. I was so exhausted and frustrated.'

Stress has many tell-tales signs, and can have its influence on just about all our normal physical, emotional and mental functions.

However, some of the clearer signs of stress are:

a   fatigue that sleep or rest does not fix
b   social withdrawal
c   flatness in mood: you feel like a washed-out dish-rag
d   muscle tension: tightness in your chest, twitching, teeth clenching, your hands restless
e   panic attacks: you have trouble breathing or you have chest pains
f   obsessive behaviour: you eat or drink too much, smoke too much, crave certain foods
g   sleep problems
h   nausea and forms of digestive problems
i   inability to concentrate
j   rumination, recurrent bad dreams.

Some of these things can have medical causes, and a doctor should be consulted in the first instance.

If the cause is not physical, there are tactics that can be employed to relieve undue stress. These include:

a   Removing the stressors: while a carer is not often at liberty to remove stressors entirely, many of the practical strategies described above can help to take some of the sting out of the situation. The aim is to reduce the causes of stress to the unavoidable ones.

b   Taking a break from the causes of stress: the old adage was that one should not run away from one's problems, but should face up to them. That may be true, but it is sometimes a matter of timing. It might be important to run away today in order to regroup and return tomorrow with a regained sense of control. This is one of the clear advantages of respite care.

c   Looking after your body: check that your diet is balanced. Give yourself opportunities for exercise, rest periods. Cut out or cut down on alcohol, smoking, caffeine.

d   Giving yourself a regular break for relaxation: relaxation techniques do not have to be highly sophisticated. A hot bath, a quiet, brisk walk in a favourite spot, a nap in front of the TV, a massage, reading a book in a park, dinner with company you enjoy, seeing a good movie are all examples of relaxation techniques. Some people find more structured activity a better course to follow. They learn meditation, they visit a church to pray or they take up yoga. Still others prefer a sporting outlet: a swim, a game of golf or tennis or bowls. Professional counsellors can teach relaxation techniques to those who are having difficulty.

e   Sharing your concerns with others: talk to a friend or family member. Perhaps you will find it easier with a minister or priest, your doctor or another professional person.

f   Seeking professional help with stress: consulting a trained counsellor or psychologist.

Conclusion

We end where we began: this is, indeed, a book about human goodness.

The people who have told their stories here are not saints or martyrs. They are ordinary people who have shown the whole gamut of human responses as they have grappled with very difficult changes in their lives. They have made mistakes and got up again. They have given in and raised themselves to extraordinary efforts.

The stories in this book are monuments to the resilience of the human spirit in the face of adversity. They speak hardly at all of doom and gloom, but mainly of the love and support found in unexpected and expected places.

We can but say thank you to the men and women who have shared their deeper feelings so that others might know that they are not alone, and that dementia does not ultimately destroy the things they value most.

Where to go for help

Information and support

If you are concerned that you or someone you know may have Alzheimer's disease, then the first thing to do is to find out as much information as you can about the disease. The Alzheimer's Association has an office in each state and provides information on the disease and advice about the services available to assist. Below is listed the Alzheimer's Association of America address and the national information hotline (toll free). The association will send information appropriate to your area upon request and will provide the telephone number of the regional Alzheimer's Association office nearest you.

Alzheimer's Association of America
70 E. Lake Street
Suite 600
Chicago, Illinois 60601-5997
Toll Free Information Hotline: (312) 853-3060

Consult your doctor

If having obtained such material you are still concerned, the next step is to consult your local doctor who may refer you to a specialist and order a number of tests. These could include a number of the following:

A CT scan of the brain;
EEG;
blood sugar, serum calcium and electrolyte tests;

serum B12 and folate levels;
thyroid and renal function tests;
microurine and culture tests;
full blood examination.

These tests are undertaken to ensure that the person does not have a reversible dementia and to obtain a comprehensive picture of the person's medical condition. Such dementias can be treated and, therefore, it is essential to diagnose correctly. The doctor may also be concerned that the person does not have symptoms similar to those of dementia but may be caused by depression. This is called pseudo-dementia. While you may feel that some of these tests are intrusive they are important in diagnosing that the dementia is irreversible. The diagnosis of irreversible dementia is one of exclusion.

Nonetheless, it is reasonable for any person receiving medical treatment to expect a clear and well-explained diagnosis. If you do not believe that your concerns are getting the attention they deserve, it is also reasonable to seek another medical opinion.

After the diagnosis

No one can deal with Alzheimer's disease on their own. The nature of the disease is such that people need support and assistance in dealing with it. In 'Stages in the progression of Alzheimer's disease' the various stages and symptoms of the disease were outlined. The nature of the support and assistance required will vary according to the stage of the disease that the person is up to. As indicated in previous sections, people often seek support and assistance too late. In the early stages, it is important to consider a number of issues:

How and when do I/we tell our family, friends and associates?

Where do I get my emotional support from?

Will we/I be able to live in this house when I am more dependent?

Do I need to set my legal and financial affairs in order?

As the disease progresses, carers often require advice about the management of difficult behaviours. It is important to know where such advice is available if you require it. Understanding that you are not alone and that others are experiencing and have experienced the same sorts of thing is often reassuring to carers. As indicated in the contributions in this book, understanding the nature of memory loss and particular communication needs of people with dementia can be helpful in assisting the person you are caring for. Being explicit with family and friends about the level and type of support and assistance you need is important. Many family members and friends want to assist but are unsure how best to. Many try to offer practical support. For some, this may be useful. For others, companionship or the chance for an uninterrupted night's sleep is most helpful. Being clear with family and friends is essential in reserving your energies for the demands of the caring role and enabling them to support you.

Susannah: Carer support groups

What's different about dementia?

Caring for a person with Alzheimer's disease is an extended and onerous task. The disease is one of slow decline and long duration. Each stage of the illness brings a new set of problems just when you think you've conquered the last.

Often it is a very confused carer who walks through the door on a first visit to a support group. Exhausted by the physical management, mentally drained by the constant creativity of problem solving and emotionally devastated by the number of losses being experienced, the carer often feels about to burst.

'I don't know who's more confused, him or me!'

Due to age, stress and grief, the carer is often in a state of poor physical and mental health. Many carers are elderly themselves yet act as the primary carer. They have to be ever vigilant, day and night. What affects one affects the other and as with a child, vibrations of joy, serenity or stress rub off. The disease may be an incurable one, but much can be done to improve the quality of life for both carer-receiver and care-giver. There is an intimate and ongoing relationship between the carer and their loved one and the carers often feel that they would be most assisted by helping the sufferer first. While the character and personality fades, the person is still there. There remains a sense of history, of a life spent together, of loyalties and love. No-one is at fault, no-one is to blame.

The unique aspect of caring for a person with dementia is the emotional destruction and isolation experienced. Carers benefit from meeting and sharing with others who are or have been in a similar situation. The strength gained in this way is quite different from support gained through other means.

'No-one can understand what it's like unless they've been through it.'

What is a carer support group?

A carer support group is a number of people who share a common need or goal, who come together voluntarily over a life-disrupting problem, for a personal change gained through mutual support.

My role as a worker with the Alzheimer Society of Victoria has been to provide resources and support to carer groups and their leaders. To assist in setting up new groups and solving problems with those established, and to encourage groups to develop skills, to grow and expand from within rather than from without.

Two-way links are maintained between the Society and the groups by use of telephone, newsletters, group visiting, seminars, consultations with group co-ordinators and putting groups in touch with each other and their local community. In this way we have together created a statewide supportive network for all carers.

How can it help?

The role of the group is one of problem solving, providing information and mutual support.

Information is the key to practical caring. Recognition of the nature of the illness helps families to know what to expect and how to manage, and provides a grounding upon which to base future decisions. It allows carers to absorb information and acknowledge new concepts at a pace in line with their emotional state. The carer is able to speak with others, find how they have coped and realise that they are not alone but in fact are in the same boat.

One member has a positive effect on another and collective problem solving and solution finding assists carers to feel less helpless, stronger, and more able to cope. The more experienced carers are able to pass on the benefit of their knowledge and experience to the newer carers and often act as a stabilising influence in the group. A bond is formed, a feeling of group solidarity develops, and confidentiality is honoured.

Feeling safe and comfortable, carers are able to express their fears, gain insight into their troubles, laugh often and cry when they need to and this results in a lowering of acute tensions and anxieties.

Group members encourage each other to maintain their independence and keep control of their lives, to accept help whenever possible, and support individual carers in the decisions they choose to make in the best interest of themselves, their families and those for whom they care.

Who better to hear it from than another who really understands?

'A problem shared in a problem halved.'

Common reasons for seeking out a support group

Carers often seek a support group in an effort to understand what is happening to their relative. Unfathomable behaviour may have been noticed for some years previously without reasonable explanation. Insidious changes in personality and character have been wiped off as part of the ageing process. They have crept into the relationship so slowly as to be imperceptible when each change occurred. Only when the carer looks back in the longer term do they realise the extent and recognise it in terms of deterioration. Finally, one day something happens so out of character or so bizarre that it no longer can be overlooked or ignored. It is at this point that help is finally sought and a diagnosis may be made.

Reeling with the implications of a diagnosis of dementia, half denying it and half believing it, the carer presents at a support group in a bewildered and shattered state.

Most of us keep private family business within the confines of the family structure and it is difficult to talk to others at first. There is a feeling of protection towards the person suffering the disease, their dignity, of not wanting others to notice the adverse change and to preserve the family unit. This may bring a reluctance to divulge the reality of the situation along with feelings of betrayal and guilt if they do. It may also leave the extended family unaware and powerless to help.

- 'I just wanted to see if others felt as I do.'
- 'I was wondering if I was doing the right thing.'
- 'Should I tell him/her that he/she has Alzheimers?'
- 'Is it genetic?'
- 'Does anyone else have trouble getting their person into the bath?'
- 'Is anyone else having this problem?'
- 'I just wanted to see if there was anything else that would 'help.'
- 'The doctor told me to come.'

Help and assistance

It is difficult for carers to accept help from outside the bounds of family and to accept it from community services may be almost unthinkable. Carers, however, need to give themselves high priority in maintaining their own health in order to care well for a relative with a dementing illness. That which constitutes help may be quite different for each of us.

The form in which community services are offered and their availability may vary from place to place. It is important to try to identify these, consider what may work best and learn before one's health runs down, to ask for assistance from the appropriate source: doctors, visiting nurses, counsellors, courses on caring techniques, the Alzheimer Society, community services, family, friends and neighbours. The support group can be of great assistance in discussing those available in the locality and they can reflect the need for support back to the reluctant carer through the examples and experiences of other members.

Carers need different types of assistance at various critical points throughout the disease. It should be matched to the behaviour or emotional response being experienced at the time. Often professional assistance can be most useful at these times.

It's perhaps the in-between times when the mutual support group can provide most assistance by maintaining approachable, regular, predictable and reliable support.

How does the group work?

The assistance gained by bringing carers together is quite distinct from that gained through other means. The power of the mutual support group lies in its sharing, numbers, acknowledgement, non-judgemental atmosphere, confidential and safe surroundings, camaraderie and accessibility to its members.

Groups acknowledge carers' loss and concentrate on 'caring' gains. They encourage each other to capitalise on what the sufferer can do and not to dwell on what they cannot, for these are lost and rarely regained. There is mutual respect for mutual problems and chances are, no matter what one's most private thought, it is likely to be shared.

'It's like lifting a heavy load off my shoulders. I feel taller after the group.'

Who leads a group, what happens, how and when and where?

All groups have leaders. Some work in the area of aged care and consider a carers' group an important part of the service they provide. Some are experienced or past carers — 'graduate carers'. Many groups may have several people who help arrange and plan group time and this can be accommodated in the self-help model. Carers develop and gain skills over time and can exercise them within the goals of the group or participate outside it through community activities. *Self-help becomes a life-style*, and there is always room for further growth. Group co-ordinators are generally very accomplished people but one can also start a support group with no prior experience.

Some groups have expanded to accommodate those who are caring for people who also have other chronic illnesses. This is usually in smaller towns to make up numbers, but none-the-less, they do work well. Some support groups are limited to special purposes. They may be carers with relatives that attend a day centre, for adult children, teenagers, spouses, men, bereavement groups or for the sufferers themselves. These are quite common in the United States.

Each group operates in its own way and has its own unique features. They may be large or small, formal or informal. All groups agree that the most important feature is mutual sharing and carer support. Priority is always given to these, so carers have the opportunity to ventilate or discuss a pressing anxiety.

Guest speakers are often invited to clarify issues or provide further information. Researchers, lawyers, financial advisors, continence nurses, supervisors from community services, specialist doctors and relaxation consultants. The group may hold educational sessions covering a wide variety of topics — stress management, pensions and benefits, preparing for residential care, patient management skills and effective group skills.

They organise social outings, keep written information and a group library, show videos, participate in public awareness campaigns and community education programs. The group co-ordinator usually has an excellent knowledge of local services and of those who are helpful and understanding in providing services.

Some groups prefer to remain as mutual sharing groups and some grow and expand their interests into broader areas. Some have developed their own initiatives. Adult day care centres, home-visiting respite care programs, a broad range of socialisation functions and fund-raising in their own local areas. One group organised their experienced carers into a 'flying squad' who made initial visits to new carers and were on call for people in crises.

Support groups commonly meet monthly for a two-hour session, at a time convenient to most. The location will be in a comfortable informal setting wherever possible, perhaps a community centre or local community building in a central location close to transport. Groups are generally free of charge, but may collect small donations for tea and coffee, etc.

New members are welcome at any time. Members may like to be regular participants or may attend only occasionally, for a variety of reasons, including transport and being unable to leave their patient.

Some groups mail a monthly newsletter which is another way to keep in touch. Some have formal 'telephone trees' where carers can call each other to chat in a difficult moment. Both act successfully as lifelines.

Group co-ordinators are available to take calls, answer queries and may meet with carers who do not wish, or are unable to attend group meetings. Family members may gain benefit from chatting on an individual basis, or wish to explore the availability of local services and other supports more privately.

There is a network of support groups throughout America; you can find the name of the contact person for the group nearest you by calling the Alzheimer's Association Toll Free Information Hotline listed on page 226.

Gains in groups

One of the great pleasures in assisting support groups and working with carers, is the privilege of seeing carers progress and take a grip on their lives as time goes by. The second is to see a whole group advance together — a miraculous change from everyone anxious to everyone rational, in perhaps twelve months or just twelve carers' meetings. This gives group members a feeling of power, enabling them to redirect their former sense of powerlessness into something positive. Group members make great celebration of these accomplishments and it provides another occasion for fun, a chance to laugh at themselves, give a pat on the back and reinforce their own progress. With time, not only do carers gain the ability to pass on this power to newer carers, but also become living examples that one *can* rebuild one's life, be indulgent in oneself again and reveal through the observation of hope that there is life with and after caring.

Support while caring at home

DOMICILIARY SERVICES

There is a range of domiciliary services available to assist you at home. Check with your local social services agency or the Alzheimer's Association to find out what is available in your area. These services are geared to enable people to live at home as long as possible. You have a right to use these services. Many are becoming more responsive to the needs of people with dementia and their carers.

While their range and level of availability differs from state to state and area to area, these services can be of considerable value in sharing the responsibilities of care. This range of services includes:

home help, for cleaning and other domestic tasks;
meals on wheels;
home maintenance, for minor household repairs;

in-home respite services, to provide someone to 'sit in' while the carer takes a break.

Your local Social Services agency or hospital can advise you of the services available in your area.

NURSING SERVICES

Nursing services provide general nursing within the home including bathing, administering of medication, dressing wounds and giving injections. Incontinence advisory services have been established in many areas. Memory loss often results in the person with Alzheimer's being unable to remember accurately the symptoms of their own ill-health. Maintenance of their general health is extremely important. The cost of these services varies according to the consumer's ability to pay. *If you want to use these services you should ask your doctor, community health center or hospital for advice about the home care nursing service in your area.*

Respite Care

DAY CARE CENTERS

Day care centers provide carers with a break from the demands of caring by allowing the person with dementia a trip outside the home. They provide interesting social programs for the person with the disease. A number of these centers have special programs for people with dementia. Staff are aware of the reluctance of people with dementia to enter a new situation and are able to assist in introducing the concept of attendance at a day care program. *Information about these centers is available from your local council, health center and hospital.*

RESIDENTIAL RESPITE CARE

Many nursing homes, hostels, geriatric centers and private hospitals provide residential care for varying periods on a short-term basis. This provides the carer with the opportunity for a break or a holiday. *Your doctor or regional Alzheimer's Association can advise you of the options available in your area.*

Permanent residential care

As the disease progresses, some people with dementia require 24-hour supervision and care. While most carers are reluctant to place someone in residential care, there often comes a point at which the carer's physical and psychological well-being can no longer take the constant demands of caring for the person with the disease. In other instances, the person becomes so frail that they are no longer able to be cared for at home. At these points, it is necessary to consider placing the person into residential care.

The type of accommodation required will depend on the degree and type of assistance the person needs.

Nursing home care will be necessary if the person needs assistance with feeding, bathing and walking and is incontinent.

Hostel care may be suitable if the person is able to feed themselves, manage their own toileting and bath and/or shower and dress with limited assistance. Medication is managed in both nursing homes and hostels.

There is a wide range of other supported accommodation facilities which offer care in the early stages of the disease. Such facilities are suitable when the person needs minimal levels of supervision and assistance.

In considering placement it is essential that you look at the facilities available in your area. You should ascertain the cost, the attitudes of management and staff to people with dementia and examine the physical features of the facility. It is generally advisable to plan one of your visits at a meal time. This provides a good indication of the realities of daily life in the facility. The decision as to where to place your loved one is an important one and it is essential to examine the options carefully.

If you experience any difficulties with the standards of care once you have placed your loved one in a nursing home, hostel or other facility for older people, first speak about your difficulties with the management of the home. There are standards which govern the quality of care and statements of the rights of residents which are generally available in printed form. Ask to see them prior to your discussion.

If you do not feel that the matter is satisfactorily resolved by talking with the management, you may like to take it further. You can contact the Department of Community Services and Health in your state, or the State Health Department.

Further reading

The following books provide information on introductory material on the disease. The Alzheimer's Association in your state can advise you of additional reading material.

Carers and caregiving

Mace, N., *The 36 Hour Day*,
Edward Arnold, 1985

A guide to the home care of those in the early and middle stages of progressive dementing illness. It combines practical advice with specific examples.

Honel, R., *Journey with Grandpa*,
John Hopkins University Press, 1988

A book rich with practical techniques and coping strategies that could be used and recognised by anyone caring for a person with dementia. It offers reassurance, and it is a moving narrative of love, faith and accommodation.

O'Connor, K. & Prothero, J., *The Alzheimer's Caregiver*,
University of Washington Press, 1987

The first part of this book addresses the nature of the disease and the second part focuses on the partner in the process: the caregiver. While the book is American it is full of pertinent facts for the carer.

Robinson, A., *Understanding Difficult Behaviours*,
East Michigan University, 1989

This publication provides some excellent advice for those caring at home and those working in residential care settings on dealing with difficult behaviours.

Gruetzner, H., *Alzheimer's: A Caregiver's Guide and Source Book*,
Wiley and Sons, New York, Brisbane, 1988
Cohen, D. & Eisdorfer, C., *The Loss of Self*,
New American Library, 1986

Incontinence

Garley, C., *Managing Incontinence*,
This book explains how the bladder works and what can go wrong and describes the many effective aids to control incontinence and make possible a normal life.

For children

Guthrie, D., *Grandpa Doesn't Know It's Me*,
Human Science Press, 1986
This is a sensitively written book for children about a young granddaughter's relationship with her grandfather who develops Alzheimer's disese. The book expresses love, understanding and the child's involvement in her grandpa's care.

Activities

Budge, Meredith, *Wealth of Experience*,
McLennan & Petty, 1989
This book provides a model structure for activities programmes and at the same time gives access to the ideas and recipes to make them work in any setting. It is a practical easy-to-read guide and best of all, it's Australian.

Zgola, Jitaka, *Doing Things*,
John Hopkins University Press, 1987
A guide to workers and volunteers who plan to carry out activity programmes within the community for persons with dementing conditions. Also an invaluable guide for individuals caring for patients at home.